THE STEALTH VIRUS

Paul D Griffiths
Professor of Virology

First published in Great Britain in 2012

ISBN: 1477566791

ISBN-13: 9781477566794

INDEX

180 million years ago- human year 2012

Prologue:
The stealth virus speaks.

"Think of a way to describe the virus that caused your last illness and I bet you'll choose words like: nasty, dreadful, abominable, poisonous and malevolent. What if I told you that I prefer the following words: beautiful, masterful, intricate and, my favourite, intelligent?

It may seem strange to you to think of a virus having intelligence. After all, we're just pieces of nucleic acid (DNA or RNA but never both) covered in a protective coat of protein and are completely inert. Until, that is, we infect somebody. Then, the information encoded within our nucleic acid instructs the human cells to stop what they are doing and start making viruses. Before each cell dies exhausted from this process of becoming a virus factory, it will have made 10,000 new daughter viruses. There are billions and billions of cells in human bodies and so there's a vast amplification of infectious material within an individual. The damage caused by the death of those cells plus the accompanying inflammation constitutes the disease that you experience. Because viruses appear in body fluids it's easy for us to transfer to someone else and repeat this infectious process in a new host. In this way, many viruses transmit from person-to-person, aided by the coughs and sneezes they produce in their victims which disseminate infected secretions into their surroundings.

But this is a precarious existence for these types of viruses because they trigger a protective immune response so that the patient can't be infected a second time. Each virus has to seek out people without such immunity and finds them in the new babies born each year. In order to survive, these viruses have to transmit very efficiently from person-to-person, which means they have to produce lots of daughter viruses very quickly, which means they have to damage lots of cells. The net result is that they cause serious disease. If a virus cannot keep transmitting to successive generations, then it dies out. The risk of this happening is increased when humans develop vaccines and encourage everyone to gain immunity without encountering the wild-type virus. You humans are likely to go to the trouble of doing this if the virus causes severe disease you can see with your own eyes. Already, I've had to watch as two beautiful viruses, smallpox and poliovirus 2, have been wiped out by you interfering humans and your wretched vaccines. To be fair, smallpox was asking for it by causing a serious rash and killing 30% of the people it infected. I had more sympathy for the 3 polioviruses, because they only caused disease in 1% of people after infecting children who were young enough to still have some protection from their mothers' antibodies. However, the disease they caused was paralysis which appeared in outbreaks among older children who had avoided infection at an earlier age. The sight of healthy young adolescents being struck down and unable to ever walk again was just too provocative for you humans to ignore, so you had to go after the polioviruses.

What if a virus was smarter; could it find a better way of persisting in the community? Yes; an intelligent virus would dodge those immune responses so that it could persist undetected within each person for years, preferably for their whole life. This would provide multiple opportunities for the virus to spread to others as each person meets new people during his/her lifetime. Because there would be multiple opportunities to transmit to others, the virus wouldn't need to produce so many copies of itself on each occasion. This means that fewer virus factory cells would be killed and so there would be fewer symptoms. We might even be able to arrange things so that there were no symptoms at all. You humans tend to keep a discrete distance from people with runny noses and coughs but, in this new situation, wouldn't know which of these carriers of the more intelligent virus was infectious. Thus, what the intelligent virus lost through not making people sneeze around others, it would gain because apparently healthy people would continue to socialise and mingle with each other, despite being infectious. The virus could then go on spreading from person-to person because it wasn't declaring its presence.

I am one of those intelligent viruses. In fact, at the risk of hubris, I'm arguably the smartest virus of our group. My family is called the herpesviruses and eight of us infect humans. You'll have heard of chickenpox, genital herpes, glandular fever and cold sores; these are diseases caused by some of the eight human herpesviruses. However, I reckon that very few of you will have heard of me, even though, if I was the product of a company, my sales penetration into the community would be the envy of the business world, because I currently infect 60% of adults in developed countries and 100% in developing countries. Well, that's just the way I like it, because I only want to persist by passing from person to person. I've no intention of drawing attention to myself by causing disease; in fact, I've spent millions of years ensuring that most people never know that I'm inside their bodies.

To give you an idea of the timescale, I've been around for hundreds of millions of years. When animals with spines started to evolve, I was there. When they started to develop immune systems I evolved with them. First, they modified the innate immunity that all living organisms possess, but I learned to deal with this. Then they developed adaptive immunity which was more sophisticated because it had memory and could remember which infections it had seen before and give an enhanced response the next time around. This adaptive immunity used white blood cells specialised into T-lymphocytes, which attacked infected cells directly and B-lymphocytes which produced soluble proteins, called antibodies, which spread in body fluids to every part of their bodies. It didn't really matter, because every time they produced a new immune weapon I developed a countermeasure.

The rate of these developments was slow, taking hundreds of years before the next one happened. This gave me or, more precisely, my ancestors plenty of time to stay in control and keep up with this arms race in immune weapons. I knew I'd always have the upper hand because nature works through evolution, creating a multitude of offspring and then selecting the one that is most fit to survive in a new situation. Because my time between generations was measured in hours, not the decades that you animals need, I was confident that I could provide offspring with improved characteristics quicker than you could.

When copying my DNA, I used careful proofreading mechanisms to maintain the authentic me. Occasionally, I made the odd mistake; most of these were fatal to my offspring but some gave an advantage and so I hung onto them. I occasionally copied a gene, kept the original to perform its intended purpose but let the duplicate change with time. Again, I hung onto those copies which helped me to co-habit the changing environment of my host and gave up those which were useless. I copied genes from the host, changed them slightly and turned them into weapons as if I was using artillery captured from the enemy. At one point, my countermeasures became too effective and allowed me to replicate so much that I started to trigger inflammation. I didn't want to give the game away by causing disease, so I copied an animal gene to damp this inflammation down. It was like an arms race, with each of us controlling the response of the other without either of us ever gaining the upper hand. Over millions of years, the immune system and I settled into a stalemate, with lots of immune cells trying to find me in the sanctuaries where I persisted, protected by my immune evasion genes.

When animals with spines set off down the pathways that would turn them into mice or men, I decided to specialise. I stuck with the big boys and said goodbye to my mousy cousin about 100 million years ago.

To illustrate how long ago that was, imagine that the branch point between mice and men was midnight on a human clock and that human year 2012 is now midnight on the next day. According to my lifespan squeezed into one day, the Romans came 2.2 seconds ago, the printing press was invented 0.57 seconds ago and the First World War started 0.1 second ago. I continued my way of life for all of these human millennia. I infected everybody and spread to every organ in their bodies, but did very little harm. I didn't need to damage cells in the process of making large numbers of daughter viruses, because I stayed with each human for all their life and had lots of chances to pass from one person to another. In particular, I learned to persist in cells of the salivary glands and kidney so that these organs secreted me to the outside in saliva and urine without getting damaged in the process. Nobody knew about me, nobody could tell I was here, nobody had treatment against me and nobody would want to make a vaccine against such an apparently innocuous infection. I had it made; I could continue my long association with the human race and transmit from person-to-person. As long as you kissed each other, I'd survive, because I'd set up home in your salivary glands. I was safe transmitting from person-to-person in secret. That's not to say I didn't have some scares over the years:

One tenth of a second ago on this imaginary 24 hour clock a problem occurred when a human learned how to perform blood transfusions. Once he realised that there were different blood groups, the procedure became safer and more common, so the few cases which transmitted me might have been seen, but I got away with it because 100% of people were infected already and so had immunity which stopped the infection giving them symptoms. My standoff relationship with the immune system stood me in good stead, because it meant I wasn't given away by producing a recognisable disease when this new medical technique was introduced.

Then, with increasing prosperity after the Second World War (0.07 seconds ago), there was an improvement in hygiene and people had smaller families. I was no longer able to infect 100% of these modern children and problems started to appear when people reached adulthood without immunity against me. Once open-heart surgery was discovered, I caused fever when fresh blood was transfused into people who weren't immune. I was worried when some prominent human you called the Pope suffered a lot by acquiring me from a blood transfusion, but the humans seemed to dismiss this as a rare case. Phew; that was a narrow escape!

I caused infection in pregnant women who hadn't acquired me when they were younger and some unborn babies died as a result. I was sorry about that, because it wasn't my intention to cause disease in the young ones who would grow up to be my host. Still, I continued to get away with it, because these cases were rare, the women didn't have symptoms to report and the doctors didn't have easy access to tests to detect me. Phew!

Then, 0.05 seconds ago some fool tried transplanting organs. My real problems started then because, by living in all organs, I was readily transmitted from the donor while the immunosuppressive drugs given routinely to transplant patients slowed down the immune system that I had carefully balanced myself against. Although I didn't want to cause disease, there was now very little to restrain me, so my full ability to replicate to high levels and cause disease was revealed. These cases were worrying, but I continued to get away with it because the transplanters were more interested in graft rejection while the infectious diseases doctors skilled in making vaccines were so focused on smallpox, polio and measles, they ignored me. Phew!

Mind you, I must admit that their vaccines have been impressive. Looking back, the first case my family or I can remember of polio was in the days of the ancient Egyptians. Later, smallpox and then measles evolved and spread widely as humans started to congregate together in towns and then cities. I had to watch as, one by one, these lovely viruses were eradicated from the globe, with measles and polio 1 and 3 just hanging on by their fingertips as I speak. This shows the folly of being a virus that has only a few days to pass from person to person if it's to survive and illustrates my superior intelligence in following a different strategy. If you humans realised that I could be controlled in the same way by vaccines then I'd be worried, but your researchers all believe that intelligent viruses like herpesviruses can never be eradicated using vaccines because we evade immune responses. They're so convinced of this that they won't even try to control me, so I'm safe for now. Phew!

About 0.05 seconds ago, human ingenuity helped a rare infection transmit from Africa to the rest of the world. You humans used your new wide-bodied jets to fly people infected with this new virus to big cities. It was called HIV and had recently crossed to humans from chimpanzees. Some of the workers on these new flying machines had lifestyles that helped them pick up new infections. After a few years of infection, HIV took away the immune system that I was pushing against and let me run wild in their bodies like I did in transplant patients. I didn't want to do it, but you interfering humans created the conditions, not me. Other infections, collectively called opportunistic, also took advantage of the lack of immunity against them and caused overt diseases, such as pneumonia. Fortunately, the doctors focused on these diseases and tended to ignore me, although I was there in nearly every AIDS patient, suppressing their immunity and spreading to every organ. Phew!

Your human ancestors were living longer because of abundant food, clean water, antibiotics and, ironically, vaccines against other viruses. If they had avoided me during childhood, they didn't transmit me when they later had their children. But, when those children had children of their own, the parents often sent them to day care centres. There, other children passed me on, so the children could transmit me to the grandparents. It wasn't my fault; these old people should have died years ago and had no right getting involved in childcare at their ages! Fortunately, these cases of disease were put down to old age, so no one recognised my contribution. I got away with it again; Phew!

Even if these older people had been infected by me in childhood, my short-term effects to divert immune responses were setting up chronic diseases once humans gained a long life expectancy. Over the years, the immune system committed more and more of its troops to attacking me, but couldn't locate all of the sanctuaries where I was hiding and so started to attack other cells instead. Some of these were in arteries so, inadvertently, I made a contribution to atherosclerosis. This disease was caused by inherited genes plus the availability of fatty foods and cigarettes, but I added to the general effect of inflammation. Again, I was lucky, because the doctors controlled the disease by reducing dietary fats and lowering blood pressure, so my contribution remained hidden because it was easier to blame diet and smoking, so I got away with it again; Phew!

These abundant, angry immune cells came to dominate as people became older and older. Doctors examining the blood of elderly people saw these groups of cells, but didn't realise that they were looking for me. The doctors didn't see that I was behind the shortage of naïve white blood cells seen in the older generation, because these cells had all been activated to chase after me living in my sanctuaries. The elderly people had difficulty responding to new infections or to vaccines because of this immune shortage. When lots of elderly people started dying from vaccine-preventable diseases like influenza, I thought I might get caught, but the doctors called all of this immunosenescence and put it down to the normal ageing process. Researchers concentrated on making better 'flu vaccines for elderly people so; once again, I escaped detection. Phew!

A sudden massive shock, such as a heart attack or tissue damage after burns stunned the immune system so that it could no longer push against me. Then I ran riot and damaged the lungs of patients, hastening their demise. In response, you humans invented intensive care units which saved the lives of many people, although the results would have been even more impressive without me. My contribution was to release cytokines which were toxic to the lungs, so leading to deaths or extended hospital care in those who survived. I worried that the doctors would take action against me, but they didn't even realise that I was there and responded by finding better ways of keeping people alive on ventilators; Phew!

Barely 0.03 seconds ago, your ancestors learned some new tricks; medical virology and molecular biology. They could discover all my clever techniques to avoid immunity and could detect me in individual people if they wanted. They couldn't keep their new insights to themselves, they told everyone about it by publishing scientific papers. They told other scientists what they had found and told them how to perform the experiments in their own labs. The legacy of the printing press from 0.57 seconds ago, updated now with rapid electronic communications, could be the end of me, especially when several prestigious Nobel prizes were awarded for work that could help to control me. Fortunately, I continued to get away with it for two reasons.

First, the scientists chose to study my mousy cousin using lots of different types of experimental mice. While this identified many of the family secrets we shared, the results could not be applied directly to humans, because the mouse and human immune systems had diverged so long ago. The impression given from decades of mouse experiments was that a herpesvirus like me was controlled solely by T-lymphocytes and could never be eradicated by vaccination. They were correct about the results of the contrived experiments they had designed in the special types of mice they had studied, but wrong about humans, so their results stopped medical researchers even trying to make vaccines against me; Phew!

Second, the physicians were still preoccupied with other diseases especially HIV, malaria and TB and didn't appreciate that, if they worked out how I persisted in humans, then some of that information could help them understand other persistent infections. Phew!

Soon after, you humans discovered a drug which was active against me and used it to treat the cases of disease which developed in patients with transplants or with HIV infection. I didn't mind this at all, because I'm not callous. I didn't intend that these cases should occur in the first place; it was you humans who damaged your own immune systems I had so carefully balanced myself against. I want to coexist with the human race and fully support your need to control the cases of disease that now occur, but what I don't support is the development of vaccines. You shouldn't throw the baby out with the bath water; you should focus on controlling disease and let me survive by passing quietly from person to person.

My plan was that you humans would continue to ignore the possibility of controlling me by vaccination like you'd always done. If not, my strategy of evolving slowly could become my Achilles' heel, because things were happening too rapidly for me to respond if I had to. For 100,000,000 years, I had kept up with slow changes, but in the last 100 years (barely 0.0001% of this time), your ancestors changed the world and evolved to become a cleaner living, longer living life form which had babies later in life, swapped organs and suppressed immune systems with drugs or with HIV. The resulting cases of disease weren't my fault; you caused them by interfering with nature and by living longer plus the unintended consequences of later pregnancies. If only the human race had continued to have a life expectancy of 25 years, then I would have had it made, but the consequences of my immunological tricks started to accumulate as you lived for decades longer. I know there are a few vaccine warriors going after me now, but I hope they won't be able to work out how vulnerable I really am. All the same, I'm getting a little worried especially when, 0.05 seconds ago, they gave me a medical name…cytomegalovirus."

Chapter 1:
1910

Almost exactly 100 years ago, histopathologists in Philadelphia recognised giant swellings within the nucleus of cells. The swellings were termed "inclusion bodies" and were so large that they made the cells appear enormous when compared to their unaffected neighbours. The histopathologists had no idea what might be causing this abnormal change to the cells, but they clearly stated that they felt it was the cause of the patient's demise.

The patient in this case had been stillborn just days before he should have been born. The obstetricians could now tell the mother that, although she had not had any symptoms during pregnancy, some strange type of infection had taken over her body, spread to her placenta and thence to her unborn baby boy. They could not tell her the name of the infection, or give any indication of whether the process might recur in a subsequent pregnancy, but simply referred to it as the *Stealth Virus*, because it seemed to slip into people's lives without anybody noticing.

Before you sweep this tragic case from your memory as an example of how primitive medical science was in those days, consider that things have not improved much over the intervening century.

Judith Jones loved children. She had babysat children since she was a teenager and now ran a small child-minding business from her own house. She had lived in the area all her life, was well known to the local mothers and got all the referrals she needed by word-of-mouth, which demonstrated that her work was well regarded. She was also flexible about timekeeping, because the business was based in her own house and so she could accommodate the needs of the professional women who used her services when they were delayed at work.

Judith would not want to be one of these mothers, because she could see how stressed they became as they rushed from work to home, trying to fit the needs of a young child into the electronic diaries which ruled their lives. No, she believed that a mother should stay at home to look after her own children at least until they were old enough to go to primary school. Of course, she never said this to any of the customers who were paying substantial sums to have their children cared for by Judith. But she did say it, repeatedly, to her husband Bert and made it clear that she would want her own baby one day. They agreed that they would try for a baby once her child-minding business was fully established.

That time came, Judith stopped taking the pill and soon told Bert one evening that he was to be a dad. They celebrated by opening a bottle of real champagne, although Judith let Bert drink most of it. As she welcomed the children the following morning, she thought that soon they would be coming to a home that had a baby of its own. She was sure she would be able to feed and look after her own little one while keeping an eye on the others. She looked forward to her expected date and, in order to reduce her workload temporarily, started to plan to not accept replacements for the two children who would soon be moving on to primary school.

All went well with the early stages of her pregnancy; the doctors told her she was healthy, the midwives did not anticipate any problems and the woman who did the ultrasound showed her a picture of her baby. Judith declined the offer of knowing whether it was a boy or a girl and took the photo home to share with Bert.

When the pregnancy was about halfway through, Judith consoled a toddler who had fallen over and received a wet sloppy kiss as he turned towards her. She didn't think any more about it, but this was the time that stealth virus came into her life for, like 40% of people, she had not been infected as a child. The virus spread silently in her bloodstream to reach all organs just like it did in everybody who was infected. But Judith was not exactly like the others, because she had a placenta which was large and full of blood as it worked to provide nutrients for her growing baby. Judith had received a lot of virus from the toddler's saliva which gave it a head start on her immune system. Although her T-lymphocytes chased after the stealth virus, they could not control it completely because they had not seen it previously and so were mounting what the doctors would call a primary immune response. The stealth virus infected cells of the placenta and grew progressively through the various layers until it infected the baby itself. The baby received a large dose of virus directly into the umbilical artery which stunned his partially developed immune system. The stealth virus spread like wildfire, gaining access to all organs and, over the course of the next two weeks, caused devastating damage to each of them.

Judith had no symptoms, because her immune system was controlling the virus; the problem was that her immunity had not been sufficient to protect her unborn baby son. All she noticed was that the baby was not kicking her as often as in the past. After a few days, she could no longer feel any kicks at all and so contacted the nice midwife who had given her the telephone number at her initial visit. She was invited to come to the hospital straight away for another ultrasound test.

The woman doing the ultrasound was not as chatty and cheerful as she had been on the previous occasion. She went off to find the midwife, who looked at the scan and then left to find one of the doctors. He repeated the ultrasound and then turned to Judith to tell her that her baby was dead. She was shocked and numb as she listened to him explain that they would induce her labour now.

They put her on the ward where other women were coming in to have their babies. As she lay on the bed with a drip in her arm administering the drug which would kick-start her uterus, she heard the lusty screams of newborn babies coming from adjacent rooms. Bert turned up to support her, but there was nothing he could say or do.

Eventually, the midwife showed Judith and Bert what they had produced. Judith held the tiny, lifeless form of the baby boy in her arms and wept uncontrollably. The midwife talked about delivering the placenta and making sure there was no bleeding, but was clinical and unemotional about it all. Once her patient was safe, the midwife helped to dry her eyes and explained that Judith had been unlucky. The baby was small and perhaps had not been meant to live. Bert said it was best for her to forget all about it and get pregnant again as soon as possible in the hope that she would be more lucky next time. Judith listened and realised that they were trying to be kind to her, but couldn't help feeling that she had failed as a mother and as a wife to Bert. She felt that it must have been her fault that the baby had died. Perhaps she was being punished by God for declining to know from the ultrasound scan whether her baby was a girl or a boy. As the midwife gently took away the dead baby, Judith heard more healthy screams from another newborn down the corridor and burst into tears again.

Looking after other people's children was not an ideal occupation for a woman who has just had a stillbirth, but Judith had no choice. The convenience of working from her own home now became a major disadvantage, as the noise and bustle of the children no longer gave her pleasure. After a week, she saw her GP and started taking antidepressant tablets. These were just beginning to work when she went back to the obstetrician to be told that an autopsy had revealed that stealth virus had killed her baby. At least she now knew what had gone wrong. She realised that she must have caught this virus from one of the children; but which one? Every time she picked up a child she wondered if this was the one who had killed her baby. If this infection was known to cause stillbirths, why hadn't the doctors made a vaccine against it to protect women like her from all this trauma?

Chapter 2:
1953-1964

The noise of popping champagne corks rang out through the normally staid coffee room in Boston. Eventually, John asked for silence and gave the speech he had been preparing for the last hour. He read out the formal letter from Stockholm which declared that Dr John Enders shared the prize for "growing polio" with his two colleagues, Drs Thomas Weller and Frederick Robbins. John was generous in his praise of these two, as well as the other researchers and support staff who had made his research successful.

He explained the terminology; what was known colloquially as the *Nobel Prize* was actually the *Nobel Prize for Physiology or Medicine*. It was awarded every year, along with prizes for chemistry, physics, literature and peace. He reminded his colleagues that the award of the prize recognised the work they had been pioneering for years in the development of cell culture. Using this technique, they had succeeded in culturing mumps virus in 1948 which would allow the culture to be developed into a vaccine. Then, in 1949 they grew poliovirus and were sure it would be worthy of publication in one of the two most prestigious journals in the world, *Science* or *Nature*. The former was based in the USA and the latter in the UK, so they decided to try *Science* to begin with. The editor sent the paper to external peer reviewers for comment on its scientific quality and importance and subsequently forwarded their opinions to the authors. John and colleagues had been delighted to read that the peer reviewers recommended that it was worthy of publication in the highly competitive *Science*.

The ability to grow poliovirus was a great breakthrough, because poliomyelitis was a serious disease which occurred in summer epidemics, striking down adolescents in particular and leaving many survivors with permanent paralysis. The public lived in perpetual fear that their strapping, healthy children might have their lives ruined, or even taken away completely, at any moment by an invisible virus. The possibility that a vaccine might now become a reality had clearly persuaded the Nobel committee to award the prize to the Harvard researchers.

Although the award of the prize meant that the Nobelists would receive many invitations to give lectures around the world, they did not slow down their research. Tom Weller, in particular, wanted to see if other viruses could be grown in cell cultures. Tom had moved to Boston to join John Enders' lab in Harvard in 1939 in order to learn this new technique of cell culture which allowed cells to be propagated and maintained for a short time outside of the body. He was keeping his eyes open for other viruses to investigate, when his 4-year old son Peter developed chickenpox.

Chickenpox infects most children, producing a characteristic rash. When the child recovers, it appears that the virus has gone away, but this is not so. The sensory nerves can become infected if the rash involves the area of skin they supply. The virus is taken up by these nerves and transported back to their base camp, called the dorsal root ganglion, situated close to the spinal cord. These cells do not divide, so the virus stays hidden there in a dormant phase, like hibernation, called "latency" for the life of the individual.

In most people, latency persists for decades because T-lymphocytes provide cell mediated immunity to suppress any attempt the virus might make to reactivate. However, cell mediated immunity tends to decline in old age in the process called immunosenescence, so that the virus eventually succeeds in reactivating in many people. It is then transported back down the nerve to produce a rash in a distinct area of skin (called a dermatome) supplied by this single nerve. This rash, called shingles or zoster, can appear anywhere on the body, but is most often found on the trunk or on the face. Because the virus often damages the nerve in the process of reactivating, patients are frequently left with chronic pain in the dermatome, even after the shingles rash has healed.

It had been known for some time that the localised rash of zoster looked similar to that of the generalised chickenpox and, in 1953, Tom had found a way of confirming this. By growing virus from cases of chickenpox (including from his son Peter) and from patients with shingles, he could compare the viruses identified in both diseases. The viruses appeared identical, showing that shingles did indeed result from reactivation of the latent form of the virus which had caused chickenpox decades earlier. This was a remarkable finding, because it showed how one virus could cause two diseases. Tom studied the virus in detail in the lab; he reported that it was a new member of the herpesvirus family and named it Varicella-Zoster virus or VZV (derived from the Latin names for chickenpox and shingles respectively).

In 1956, Tom grew another virus from the liver biopsy of a child and gave it its name, cytomegalovirus, or CMV for short, because it made cultured cells swell up (cytomegaly = large cell). Two other laboratories had also grown CMV independently. They all reported that it was another member of the herpesvirus family, like chickenpox, so the mid-1950s were a good time for discovering herpesviruses.

Just like Tom had done following the discovery of his other viruses, the availability of this new virus in cell cultures allowed him to develop tests to measure whether individuals had made antibodies against CMV. These studies revealed that infection with CMV was common; 60% of adults had been infected, rising to 100% among the sections of the population residing in poorer areas where infections were readily transmitted within large families. People with antibodies were termed seropositives, whereas those without antibodies were called seronegatives. Clearly, CMV was transmitted from person to person, but what symptoms did it cause? How serious was it? Would it be worthwhile making a vaccine against CMV in the way that his research had led the way for vaccines against other viruses? Tom decided to continue searching for new viruses while helping to develop vaccines against the four he had already isolated.

Soon, it was time for another member of Tom's family to help with his research. Ten-year old Robert Weller became ill with a fever and a rash which was typical of German measles, so Tom was relieved that his son did not have a serious illness. He also saw a scientific opportunity and collected some samples of throat swab, blood and urine to see if he could grow this virus in cell cultures. He kept the cells going for as long as possible and eventually saw signs of damage on the cells inoculated with Robert's urine which might represent the effects of the virus; its *cytopathic effect*. To differentiate this possibility from some non-specific toxic effect of the urine on cells, Tom passed the fluid from one set of cells on to another. If it was a toxic effect it would disappear as the urine was diluted in the culture fluid, but if it was a virus replicating in the cells, then it would still be there despite dilution. Eventually, he saw the same tell tale signs in serial sets of cells and concluded that he had indeed cultured rubella to claim his fifth human virus!

This first culture of rubella was important, because it provided the possibility that a vaccine might be made against this virus. Tom's track record of achieving this for mumps and polio stood him in good stead, so he decided to repeat the process for rubella. This disease in adults and children was insignificant, as illustrated by Robert's rapid recovery. Some adult women got painful joints following rubella which persisted for weeks or months, but that minor disability would not on its own justify creating a vaccine and giving it to all children. However, rubella did have a dark side for, if a woman contracted it during pregnancy, she could have a baby whose heart, ears or eyes were damaged. This phenomenon had been described by an ophthalmologist in Australia and was about to be demonstrated on a grand scale in the USA.

Rubella occurs in spring-summer epidemics and the one of 1964 was bigger than most. The people at greatest risk were women in the first third of their pregnancies, when the fetal organs are in the process of forming. Add the additional 6-7 months of gestation to a spring-summer epidemic and one can see why a large number of women delivered babies damaged by rubella around Christmas time 1964. This abundance of cases, and their presentation around the traditional moment of family togetherness, triggered a strong response among the US population, who generously gave money to support the

March of Dimes. This charity had been established after Franklin Roosevelt contracted polio as an adult. Although paralysed from the waist down, he ran successfully for President of the USA without the press ever discussing his disability; showing that a wheelchair was not a barrier to high office. The charity used its funds to provide practical help to people damaged by polio and also to support research towards a vaccine. The latter had been so successful that the charity was delighted to support development of another vaccine against a virus which also caused disability. So, Tom's discovery of how to grow rubella virus in the lab was applied rapidly to develop a vaccine.

Tom could now follow the results as vaccines were developed clinically against 3 of the 5 viruses he had identified. What about the fourth and fifth? In particular, Tom wondered whether the same principles pioneered to prevent rubella causing damage to developing babies could be applied to CMV, which was known to damage the fetus, although it affected the brain and hearing predominantly, sparing the heart and (usually) the eyes which were both damaged by rubella. He encouraged his new research fellow, Charles Alford, (known to everyone as Charlie), to focus on CMV and ways of growing it in the lab which were based on cultures of fibroblast cells. CMV was a real pain to work with in the lab because, like rubella, it took a long time to produce cytopathic effect, but Tom had a few strains which grew better in the lab and so they could plan the first experiments. Charlie proved to be a skilled and enthusiastic researcher, although his Alabama accent was difficult to understand sometimes. This got him teased by his new colleagues in Harvard, who all had clipped East Coast accents.

In Colorado, a pathologist was writing up the autopsies on patients who had failed to survive renal or liver transplantation; a new treatment which was literally life saving in some people, yet hastened the death of others. Patients had to be given immunosuppressive drugs to stop their T-lymphocytes rejecting the graft, but the drugs available were crude. The doctors felt they were walking a tightrope with irretrievable graft rejection leading to death as one effect of not enough immunosuppression and life-threatening opportunistic infections as an effect of too much. In both cases, patients often had fever, so it was difficult to be sure which pathological process had the upper hand at any one time in an individual patient. The results of full autopsies would provide important information which they could apply to the management of their next patients.

A total of 61 transplants had been performed at the pioneering Colorado Centre and 32 had come to autopsy. The results of the examinations showed that CMV was rife among their tissues, with the characteristic inclusion bodies, which had first been seen in 1910 in a case of stillbirth, being seen regularly in the lungs as well as in the transplanted organ. In most cases, the transplant had been successful but the patients had died from complications, particularly pneumonia and, among the infections causing pneumonia, CMV was top of the list. The results needed to be known widely, so the authors prepared the technical descriptions for publication. Just as *Science* and *Nature* are the foremost journals publishing scientific research, so the *New England Journal of Medicine* and the *Lancet* are the major medical journals. The former is based in the USA and the latter in the UK, so the authors decided to send the paper to the *New England Journal of Medicine* in the first instance. The peer reviewers agreed that the article contained such important information that it was worthy of publication in the prestigious *New England Journal of Medicine* as a warning that CMV was holding back the development of this new treatment and that doctors should err on the side of keeping doses of immunosuppressive drugs as low as possible.

Harry Collins was not healthy, despite his young age of 20. He had spent much of his life attending hospital to have his liver function measured and was getting worse not better.

"I'm sorry Harry, but we've come to the end of the list of things we can offer you here."

"What's going to happen to me now?"

The doctor thought for a moment, choosing his words carefully:

"Your blood is being poisoned, because your liver isn't working properly. The poisons are slowly building up in your body."

"I know that, because you've told me many times; but what's going to happen next?"

The doctor hated doing this, especially when the patients were so young:

"You'll feel more and more sick, then sleepy. We'll make you comfortable with some medicine."

"You mean I'm going to die? You can't just let me die! Isn't there something else I can do?"

The doctor thought for a moment; he didn't want to give his patient false hope, but Harry was so young that he might be able to become one of the survivors of the new technique everyone was talking about.

"The University of Colorado has an experimental program to take a liver from one person and transfer it into another. It's called transplantation, but is very risky. I think about half of the patients don't survive the process."

"Half a chance is better than none at all. How do I get to Colorado?"

The view from his bedroom window showed snowcapped mountains, but Harry couldn't enjoy the vista. The doctors had told him about all the risks and he was to be given a last chance at life now that someone had been killed in a road traffic accident. Harry took one last look out of the window as the man wheeled the gurney out of his room.

When Harry came round, he couldn't work out where he was. Was this heaven?

"Hello Harry; your throat will be sore, because of a tube we needed to put down to help you breathe. Would you like a sip of water?"

Harry couldn't speak, but nodded to the nurse who cushioned his head to let him draw cool water through a straw. The water was refreshing, but the effort required to get it was so exhausting that he fell back asleep.

Harry woke to hear two doctors talking about him as if he wasn't there.

"The bilirubin is rising again so we'd better give another dose of steroids."

"Are you sure? The last patient we did that to got stealth virus and ended up downstairs."

"I know, but we'll lose the liver if we don't do anything."

Harry drifted in and out of sleep, but then got a cough. It got worse until he fell asleep for the last time.

In the autopsy room downstairs, his lungs were found to be full of inclusion bodies.

"We've got to find a way of knowing which patients have this stealth virus. If only there was a test for it, we could hold off on the steroids."

"What if they then rejected the liver?"

"We'd have to give them a second one," said the surgeon. "I'm not going to give up on this program, but we've got to do better than we're doing now."

Chapter 3:
1965–66

It was snowing in Helsinki when a 33-year-old man was admitted to Aurora Hospital with fever and headache. Laboratory tests showed abnormal liver function tests and "atypical lymphocytes" in the blood. A clinical diagnosis of infectious mononucleosis was made, which was also known as glandular fever.

Infectious mononucleosis is a syndrome that can be caused by several different infectious agents. Many people with this condition have antibodies in their blood which stick to sheep red blood cells. This odd phenomenon is used as a diagnostic test and is usually positive in people whose lymph nodes are swollen and who have sore throats. The man in Helsinki had neither of these clinical features and his blood did not react with sheep red blood cells.

Intrigued, the doctors looked out for more cases of infectious mononucleosis and collected a series of 14; 9 with sore throat and positive sheep red blood cell test and 5 with neither feature. They wondered if any of these cases was caused by a virus which had only recently been described and included CMV in their search. They had received strains of this virus in 1959 from the USA and had grown it up in the lab to make enough material to create a test for antibodies against CMV.

All 5 patients with the unusual form of infectious mononucleosis had no antibodies to CMV when they presented with their illnesses, but all 5 promptly made these antibodies over the next two months. This pattern was not seen in any of the 9 patients who had the typical form of infectious mononucleosis with sore throat, swollen lymph nodes and antibodies that reacted with sheep red blood cells. The authors, led by Dr Leevi Kaariainen, concluded that CMV was the cause of this unusual type of infectious mononucleosis and wrote a paper in the *British Medical Journal* saying so.

The following year, Dr Kaariainen sent another paper to the *British Medical Journal.* It was known that some patients developed a fever about a month after open heart surgery. The fever typically lasted 2 to 3 weeks, "atypical lymphocytes" were found in the blood and the test for antibodies that stick to sheep red blood cells was negative. This syndrome looked just like the cases of infectious mononucleosis that the doctors had seen, so they looked for CMV antibodies using their new lab test.

All 3 patients who had this syndrome made antibodies to CMV promptly after receiving fresh blood, so the doctors concluded that this was the cause of the previously mysterious syndrome.

Alice Kirby was a bright girl. She had just completed the first year of her two-year A-level studies in English, French and History and was predicted to get A-grades in all three. She was an only child whose parents doted on her. In particular, her father, who was a low-level civil servant, exhorted her repeatedly to succeed academically so that she could have a better life than him. Alice was diligent with her studies and was fully determined to follow her father's advice. She was very happy at school and had recently found a boyfriend.

Philip was in her year at school. They were both studying English and French, although Geography was his third subject. They started out by sharing teaching notes and discussing their set books. It was convenient to read these books together sitting outside in the fresh air and the past summer had certainly been hot. Their relationship blossomed and they spent some evenings together going to the cinema and sitting in the back row kissing. Philip wanted to go further, but Alice would have none of it. She was absolutely determined to follow her father's advice and establish her academic credentials by getting straight A-grades. She did enjoy kissing Philip though.

They compromised by allowing themselves occasional evenings off from their studies while planning to go to the same university where Alice would at last go on the pill and have a full relationship away from the all-seeing eyes of her parents. Meanwhile, Alice's pent-up adolescent sexual desires were requited by regular trips to that back row of the cinema.

Philip had acquired the stealth virus as a toddler and so was part of the 60% of the population who were seropositive. He was not permanently infectious to others because the virus spent most of its time in a latent form, hiding away from the immune system in various sanctuary sites within every part of his body. From time to time it reactivated from these sanctuaries to become infectious, so any of his organs or any body fluid could transmit stealth virus to someone else. Philip's teenage brain was thinking about a body fluid he would like to share with Alice, but she had made it clear that there was no chance of that until they went to university. Another site of latency which stealth virus could reactivate from was his salivary glands. While not watching a film she had paid to see, Alice acquired stealth virus from Philip and got a large dose because she spent so long enthusiastically sharing his saliva.

Alice belonged to the 40% of people who had not been infected with stealth virus in the past and so was destined to have a severe illness from the quantity of virus she had been challenged with. Six weeks later, Alice was struck down with a sudden high fever and debilitating malaise. She could not raise her usual enthusiasm for anything and, for the first time in years, stayed in bed instead of going to school. Her mother was so concerned at this unusual behaviour that she phoned to get a doctor's appointment. He confirmed that Alice had a raised temperature and told her she had glandular fever, caused by a virus which made cytokines circulate around her body. He told her that one causative virus had recently been identified, but that others could produce similar symptoms. The treatment was the same for all of them, so he took some blood for diagnostic tests and advised her to rest, drink clear fluids and take paracetamol to reduce her fever.

The treatment had little effect and Alice remained completely wiped out. Her mother was concerned about her health while her father added that Alice needed to keep on top of her studies. The doctor reported that Alice had glandular fever caused by stealth virus, that it had affected her liver and that it could take weeks to resolve. He advised continuing with rest, fluid and paracetamol.

Alice remained virtually bedbound and missed many lessons. She responded to her father's encouragement to keep on top of her reading, but kept falling asleep, even if her mother moved her out into the sunny garden. Philip helped her make the application for the university they planned to attend together, but was shocked at her loss of drive and beauty. Her debility continued in this way for the whole of the Autumn term although she started to improve just as school was closing down for the Christmas holidays. In the New Year, she was able to go back to school, but remained weak and had lost some of her determination and enthusiasm. She also felt that her memory was not as good as it had been. She saw Philip at lessons and he helped her with revision, but they never went to the cinema again. Alice studied as hard as she could, but knew that she was just a pale version of her previous self.

This subjective assessment was confirmed by her objective marks in the A-levels when she received two D grades and one C grade. This was not sufficient for her to go to the good university that had made her a provisional offer, so she reluctantly accepted the advice of her teachers that she should repeat the year and apply to university in 12 months' time, citing her major medical problem in mitigation. Alice's father wondered if the doctors realised the havoc that this virus had wreaked on his daughter, and thousands of teenagers like her, and wondered why they hadn't made a vaccine to protect against what seemed to be a common problem.

Philip got two A grades and one B grade, so meeting the criteria laid down in his provisional offer. He said goodbye to her as he set off for the University that he and Alice had planned to attend together. Within days of the start of Freshers' Week, he would share his saliva and that other precious body fluid he had longed to be rid of with another student who would subsequently join Alice in failing to get the grades she deserved.

Chapter 4:
1971-1975

Tom Weller had spent more time working on CMV than any other investigator. He knew the few people who had tried to research this difficult area and had sent many of them strains of virus which grew much better than those isolated directly from patients; the wild-type virus. By 1971, he felt it was time to summarise current knowledge about this virus and submitted a review to the *New England Journal of Medicine*. It was a tour de force and gave many perspectives which warned contemporary researchers not to over-interpret their data or to ignore the clinical effects of congenital CMV.

For example, he counselled against the common practice of sharing between labs a particular strain of CMV which grew much more easily than did strains collected directly from patients. While this strain was easier to work with, Tom warned that it might have acquired genetic changes to allow better growth in the lab and so might no longer fully represent the authentic CMV circulating among humans. Tom also emphasised that CMV was a much greater threat to developing babies than was rubella, because of the sheer number of cases. Rubella made an impact because it occurred in epidemics from time to time when many women developed a rash and sought medical care. In contrast, CMV silently infected women year in, year out; they could not seek advice, because they were not aware that they had a problem. Looking back over the past seven years, Tom counted about 500 cases of congenital rubella in the USA compared to over 10,000 cases of congenital CMV.

In Japan, Dr Michiaki Takahashi looked at the three-year-old boy called Oka who had chickenpox. Dr Takahashi had infected cell cultures in his lab from this boy and had decided to develop a vaccine against chickenpox. He looked after children with leukaemia and had seen several die when they encountered VZV for the first time, because the drugs needed for their leukaemia treatment damaged their immune systems. These human tragedies were bad enough, but the knowledge that he had cured most of the children of their leukaemias only to see them succumb to chickenpox drove Dr Takahashi to do something about it. He took the virus he isolated and kept it growing in the lab by passing it repeatedly from one set of cell cultures to another. Just as a virus acquires mutations which help it adapt to humans when it passes from person to person, so the opposite happens when strains are selected to grow best in cell cultures. Passing a virus in serial cell cultures had become the standard way of preparing prototype vaccines. Eventually, he ended up with a strain which looked as if it was mild enough to be ready for trial in humans and called his vaccine strain *Oka*.

It is fair to say that Dr Takahashi's plans were controversial. Because patients being given cancer chemotherapy have damaged immune systems, it is forbidden to give them live vaccines; even if the strains are mild in normal people, they may still cause serious disease in those who are immunocompromised. Dr Takahashi avoided this problem by taking advantage of the ways that courses of intensive chemotherapy were given to children, followed by weeks of no treatment in between. He let the children's immune systems recover partially and then gave the live *Oka* vaccine before they received their next course of intensive chemotherapy. In 1974, his results were published in the *Lancet*, one of the two top journals dealing with medical research.

After his training in the Harvard lab, Charlie Alford had returned to his native Alabama and established a research group in Birmingham. He recruited two bright research paediatric fellows of his own, Sergio Stagno, newly arrived from Chile and Rich Whitley, a graduate of the prestigious Duke Medical School. Charlie encouraged the former to focus on defining the natural history of CMV infection and the latter on evaluating the new field of antiviral therapy; conventional wisdom said that it was impossible to make drugs against viruses, but that was all about to change.

Sergio analysed the results of a long and painstaking natural history study. In babies with congenital rubella, the isolation of virus proved that the disease in a baby with heart malformations had been caused by rubella. Yet, the same appeared not to be true for CMV. He collected urine samples from all babies born at local hospitals. Using the new technique of cell culture which Charlie had brought back from Boston and established in the Alabama lab, Sergio could identify babies born with congenital CMV infection and examine them carefully to describe the full clinical effects caused by this virus.

However, only a minority of babies born with CMV in their urine had symptoms. True, several of them were seriously damaged, but the majority appeared to be normal at birth. Some of these children developed symptoms later, especially suffering from hearing loss as they grew older. It was a special type of hearing loss, not caused by the build up of fluid in the middle part of the ear, known as glue ear, which could be treated by the insertion of tiny drainage tubes. Instead, it was a type of damage to the nerves in the inner ear. This type, called sensorineural hearing loss, often got worse with time and there was no known treatment. Yet, most babies born with CMV appeared to be normal. Why did some get disease while others escaped? Was the new test for culturing CMV in cell cultures too sensitive, in that it was picking up mild cases of congenital infection with no clinical significance? Was it the children with the greatest burden of virus who got disease? Sergio had decided to investigate these possibilities by not just culturing each urine sample but making several dilutions of it and inoculating each dilution independently into cell cultures. This was tedious, expensive and laborious work for his technical staff, but would indicate which children had lots of virus, because it would still be detectable even when their urine was diluted, and which had only a small amount of virus. He linked together the results showing the quantity of virus in the urine collected at birth with the results from the clinical follow-up of the same children and looked at the combination.

The amount of CMV in the urine was very high in some children and much less in others, so he had to calculate the logarithm of the quantity in order to be able to plot the results on a single piece of graph paper. Once he had done this, the interpretation was fairly clear-cut. Children who did not have congenital CMV infection, but acquired it at birth through breast-feeding, never got disease and the results confirmed his guess that they had a low quantity of CMV. The second group were babies with congenital CMV who so far had not developed any symptoms. They had more virus than the previous set of babies, about 10 times as much, so he plotted their results as having one extra unit of CMV on his logarithmic scale. The last group of babies were those with congenital CMV in whom the virus had caused damage. These had about 10 times as much again virus in their urine, or 100 times that found in the first group, so he plotted their results as one extra logarithmic unit above the second group. The results on the graph showed that, unlike rubella, many babies escaped damage when they were infected with CMV in the uterus. The ones who suffered were those who had lots of virus at birth.

As part of Sergio's study design, the technical staff had diluted all the urines that came from these children when they attended the follow-up clinics. He next turned his attention to these results. Remarkably, all children carried on having CMV in their urine for years, but the quantity dropped off rapidly; by the time they were six months old, the values from those with symptoms were no different from those without. This showed that large amounts of CMV damaged the developing fetus and continued to do so for a few months after birth, which might be why some babies developed hearing loss later when their hearing had definitely been normal at birth. This was quite unlike rubella, where all the damage was done while the baby's organs were developing during the first third of pregnancy.

Sergio performed statistical tests on these results and wrote them up into a detailed scientific paper. It turned out to be a classic, because it showed that what was later called the viral load was important for CMV; the first time that this had ever been shown for any virus that infected humans. Put simply, the more virus that was present, the worse the disease. Sergio did not know this, but the measurement of viral load would, decades later, become a standard way of monitoring patients with infections like HIV (which, unbeknown to everyone, had already crossed from chimpanzees to humans and was at that time in the process of transmitting slowly from person to person in Africa).

In London, Paul Griffiths was a medical student with an interest in viruses who had been taken under the wing of the Professor of Virology, Raymond Heath and given a project on a newly discovered infection called serum hepatitis while he chose a virus to focus on for long-term research. As Paul read about all the viruses which affected patients, he came across a case of CMV and looked up in textbooks what was known about it. Having consulted two large tomes he was dissatisfied with the result, because there was little information about CMV itself and most of the discussion appeared to be extrapolated from what was known about other viruses, especially rubella. The textbooks dismissed CMV as a puny thing which only rarely caused any medical problems and then only in patients whose immunity was suboptimal, such as the developing fetus or transplant patients given large doses of drugs to stop their immune systems rejecting their new organs. This impression of a puny virus was reinforced by the behaviour of CMV in the lab, for it took weeks to grow in cell cultures in contrast to important pathogens like polio which destroyed similar cells within days.

Paul reasoned that this did not make sense. If transplant patients were immunocompromised they should suffer from the most aggressive viruses, not just the puny ones. It made more sense for CMV to be normally controlled effectively by a brisk immune response so that it would only appear clinically once drugs were given to suppress immunity, or when immunity had not fully developed in the case of a fetus. If this were true, it meant that the examples of CMV grown in cell cultures in the lab were giving the false impression of a puny virus, perhaps because the fibroblasts were the wrong cell line or because the lab-adapted strains of CMV were not representative of the virus which infected humans. He then came across Tom Weller's 1971 review article and was impressed by the way this Nobel Laureate admitted and drew attention to gaps in knowledge about CMV instead of trying to pretend that he understood everything about this virus. Paul decided to follow Weller's advice that we should be guided by evidence, not by suppositions. Paul dismissed the glib descriptions given in the textbooks and coined the phrase: *the wrong virus in the wrong cell line using the wrong end point* to describe the conventional approach of studying laboratory adapted strains of CMV in fibroblast cell cultures by means of their cytopathic effect.

A study had just been reported from St George's Hospital, also in London, of detecting primary CMV infection in pregnant women by measuring the appearance of antibodies, so Paul decided to extend these results by testing more patients. Professor Heath's virology lab already received blood samples from women in the early stage of pregnancy to test for antibodies against rubella, so he just had to get permission to collect another sample at delivery and could then see who had become infected by the appearance of antibodies against CMV, using the test developed in Helsinki. Paul had identified the virus he wished to focus his research on and reasoned that, if it was deemed important to control congenital rubella by means of vaccination, then Tom Weller's results showed it would definitely be worthwhile doing the same for CMV because this virus caused much more disease than did rubella. He should just have time to complete this study before he had to concentrate on taking his final medical exams, but thereafter aspired to focus on a career in medical virology and help take CMV from obscurity to elimination.

His early results from the study of pregnant women were subtly different from those published earlier from the other part of London. He found that the infection was common, but that only one third of women transmitted CMV to their fetus, not the 50% implied by the earlier study. This difference might seem small mathematically, but it would make a major difference when counselling a patient that her risk was 33% instead of 50%. Paul had been taught not to give risks in percentages, because many members of the general public were more familiar with the odds that they could obtain from bookmakers, so he described the risks as 1 in 3 instead of 1 in 2, although it would take a few more years before there were enough cases to be certain of the true value. The lack of hard data about this virus convinced Paul that CMV was the virus on which he should focus.

It seemed ironic that the researchers had derived the *mega* part of its name from *large* whereas they allocated this apparently mild virus only a *small* part of their textbooks on medical virology. He noticed that many of the published papers came from Alabama and asked Professor Heath if he would enquire if Paul could visit their lab for his elective in the following year. Professor Heath wrote to Charlie and received an enthusiastic response that they would be pleased to see Paul.

Fred Hutchinson was a famous baseball player who died from a nasty neurological disease. His brother raised funds to create a research institute in his name in 1975 in Seattle and settled on the development of bone marrow transplantation as the subject of clinical research to be pursued.

Pioneering work by Dr. E. Donnall Thomas in dogs and then humans would win him the *Nobel Prize for Physiology or Medicine* in the future for showing that this procedure was possible. A team of people would now try to bring the theory into routine clinical practice for humans. Essentially, they would use drugs to poison the patient's bone marrow so that they created "room" for new bone marrow to be taken up once it was infused. The drugs were very toxic, so their administration could only be justified if the patient had a life-threatening disease. Why not choose a disease of the bone marrow for which these drugs were prescribed already? So, the plan was to take patients with leukaemia, treat them with toxic drugs at such high doses that they killed the cancer and then irradiate the bone marrow in addition. The damage to the bone marrow would then be repaired by fresh bone marrow taken from a brother or sister.

If the patient was lucky enough to have an identical twin, then the procedure could be relatively safe. But, if not, there was a risk that the new marrow would recognise the patient's tissues as being foreign and cause graft versus host disease. This could be controlled with immunosuppressive drugs like steroids, but these patients were immunosuppressed already and so would be at extreme risk of opportunistic virus infections. These viruses could come from outside the patient or, if the patient had a latent virus onboard when they came into hospital, this virus could reactivate once the immune system keeping it under control was removed. In the case of CMV, the problem was reactivation of latent virus.

Julie Jefferies was a bubbly 19-year-old brunette who worked in a bakery shop. She was friendly to all the customers and was liked by all who knew her.

One afternoon, she began to feel tired and then lethargic. She struggled through her shift, but went to bed early as soon as she got home. Her mother was so concerned about this unusual situation that she made Julie stay in bed the next morning and telephoned their family doctor. Julie struggled to the surgery that afternoon accompanied by her mother. The doctor noticed that Julie looked pale, so took some blood tests and advised her to go back to bed.

The haematology technician working the evening shift was concerned by the excess of white blood cells. He made a thin film on a glass slide from Julie's blood, stained it and looked under the microscope. He had seen the pattern before, so telephoned the consultant haematologist:

"We have a new case of acute lymphoblastic leukaemia. I'll leave the slides for you to look at tomorrow morning."

At 8 AM, the consultant reviewed the slides, confirmed the diagnosis and telephoned the GP:

"I'm afraid your patient Julie Jefferies has acute lymphoblastic leukaemia. Please send her to the ward today for additional blood tests and bone marrow examination."

Julie was stoical through all the tests. They discussed the options with her and her mother went home to ask her son Jeremy if he would donate bone marrow to try to save the life of his sister. Normally, Jeremy would be teasing his younger sister but, instead, gave her a long hug as he volunteered to do anything to bring her back to health. Julie reviewed the pros and cons of the possible treatments with the doctors once again before opting for bone marrow transplantation. She started chemotherapy the next day and her count of abnormal white blood cells came plummeting down. She was next sat in front of a linear accelerator to receive a dose of x-rays to destroy her bone marrow. Normally, this dose would be as lethal as that received at Nagasaki or Chernobyl, but the doctors planned to rescue her bone marrow with an infusion from Jeremy.

Within a month of first feeling ill, Julie watched as her brother's bone marrow ran out of a plastic bag down a tube and into a vein in her arm. A few days later, Julie developed a sore mouth that was so painful that the doctors gave her morphine mouthwash. She then developed a fever and felt lightheaded, but the doctors resuscitated her with fluid and antibiotics. They explained that bloodstream infections with bacteria were common when patients were short of white blood cells. How ironic that she had come into hospital because she had too many white cells and was now ill because she didn't have enough.

Eventually, they told her that Jeremy's bone marrow had engrafted within her, so that the white cell count in her body was starting to increase. Within 3 weeks of the transplant, she had enough white blood cells to protect her from bacterial infections. She was feeling much better and could see the light at the end of the tunnel, now that Jeremy's white blood cells were working on her behalf.

Unfortunately, just as Jeremy teased Julie, so the lymphocyte component of his white blood cells attacked his sister, causing a rash, fever and diarrhoea as part of graft versus host disease. Having been better for a few days, Julie now felt dreadful. The doctors gave her steroids which suppressed the rash and the diarrhoea somewhat.

Jeremy's T-lymphocytes were acting like a two-edged sword. They were causing graft versus host disease to make her ill, but were also preventing latent stealth virus in Julie's body from reactivating. Once the doctors gave Julie steroids, these drugs knocked out the T-lymphocytes to reduce the graft versus host disease, but also reduced their ability to control stealth virus. Nothing happened for a week, but then this virus appeared in her blood and kept increasing in quantity. Eventually, the viral load in her blood overwhelmed the natural barriers that stop viruses gaining access to organs. In her case, the virus went to her lungs.

Julie could hardly catch her breath. The doctors moved her to the intensive care unit and soon had to put a tube in her neck to pump air directly into her lungs. She was sedated to allow this to happen, so was a sorry sight when Jeremy and their mother visited that evening.

Julie's brave fight came to an end 10 days later when her lungs had been damaged so much that oxygen was no longer reaching her brain. Julie's mother had to make the agonising decision to switch off the machines that were keeping her daughter pink, although the doctors insisted that she wasn't sleeping, but was brain-dead.

At autopsy, the doctors confirmed that Julie had died from stealth virus pneumonia and commented that her leukaemia had been cured.

Chapter 5:
1976-1981

The purpose of an elective period abroad is to let students have two months to experience how health care is practised in other countries. Most students tacked their four weeks' annual holiday on to their elective period and Paul was no exception; he planned to spend three months in the USA, mostly in Alabama learning about CMV. The cheapest way to get there was to fly with a budget airline from London to New York, followed by Greyhound bus to travel the approximately 1,000 miles from New York to Alabama. The bus company offered an open ticket which allowed as many journeys as could be fitted into seven days, so Paul bought one as a way of exploring a country he had never visited before. He had also never flown on a plane, but the McDonnell Douglas DC10 was a superb introduction when the time came. The plane was enormous when viewed from the departure area at Gatwick airport and instilled great confidence that both it and he would survive the transatlantic journey.

After exploring New York City from a cheap hotel in the lower east side for two days, Paul located the bus terminal and decided on the destination of his first trip on a Greyhound.

He had seven days to get to Alabama and took in as many cities as possible on an ambitious itinerary, visiting Philadelphia, Cleveland, Chicago, St Louis, Oklahoma City, Little Rock and then finally Birmingham Alabama. The bus stopped during the night at intermediate cities and provided examples of how the poorest sections of communities lived and travelled; more akin to a Third World country than to one of the world's two superpowers. He mused it was clear how infections could flourish in such circumstances, leading to a greater burden in the people with least resources, illustrating why CMV could be so common in some parts of the country.

The public displays at each city gave a better history lesson than any he had received at school. 1976 was bicentennial year and Paul enjoyed looking at all of the local history which schoolchildren had assembled, once he got used to the new terminology. What he had been taught was the *American Revolution* was termed the *War of Independence*. The local people he thought of as *revolutionaries* had been *freedom fighters*. He enjoyed reading about how beastly the British had been to the new Americans and how mad King George had mismanaged the inevitable process of democratisation. Furthermore, when he reached the deep South, he heard that a later conflagration, the *American Civil War*, was called the *War of Northern Aggression*. Clearly, history was not an objective subject, but one which was subject to revision from the perspective of the observer.

As Paul was leaving New York, something else was arriving in the city to take part in the celebratory atmosphere. The virus we now call HIV had relocated from Africa courtesy of airline travel. This new visitor would not declare its presence for another five years, but would have a profound effect on the public and the subject of medical virology.

Paul was welcomed into the Alabama lab and told that he had arrived at a busy, but opportune, time. The five-year grant which provided their funding was up for renewal and a series of speakers were preparing what they would present to the visiting scientists who made up the site review committee. Paul sat at the back of the lecture theatre to enjoy a series of state-of-the-art lectures and listened intently as they anticipated what questions might be asked and practised suitable answers. It was a wonderful introduction to CMV, because each speaker provided background information about his/her topic as well as new, unpublished, scientific data.

Sergio summarised his results showing that babies with the highest viral load were those destined to develop disease. Paul was interested in pathogenesis, that is, understanding the ways that viruses cause disease and wanted to follow up the implications of the study when he got back to London. He would have to design a new laboratory method, which would be a good topic for his research thesis as part of his training in medical virology. The implications were that CMV was growing in all parts of the body. He couldn't gain access to study it in the inner ear or the brain, but could measure it in the urine. By collecting serial samples of urine, he could potentially monitor what was going on in the inaccessible organs being damaged by CMV. Given his concerns about the virus grown in cell culture not being representative of the real thing, this monitoring should be done using a method that did not require cell cultures. The results must be quantitative, so that responses to any antiviral treatment (if one was discovered in the future) could be assessed. Indeed, the fact that the viral load was only higher for a few months after birth implied that relief from progressive disease might be obtained with short term therapy, which would be much easier to tolerate than treatment which had to be continued for years. At that time, there were no licensed antiviral drugs, but it was hoped that they could be developed in the future. Sergio's results also showed that CMV was different from the other known herpesviruses. While they could reactivate from time to time, for example when latent VZV awakened in sensory nerves to cause shingles, CMV set up a persistent, chronic infection in these young babies. This observation implied that an immune deficit specific for CMV was induced and it would be illuminating to know how this was achieved.

Sergio next described the results of a study showing that women who were immune to CMV before they became pregnant could nonetheless deliver babies congenitally infected with CMV. This was completely against the dogma which Paul had read in the textbooks and completely unlike rubella. When challenged, Sergio explained that the textbooks had merely stated (or overstated) an opinion that CMV would follow the example of rubella without providing any evidence to support this. The results he was describing came from the first study designed to test this assumption directly and would revolutionise the way people thought about CMV. Paul concluded that the study he was doing in the London lab in pregnant women with primary CMV infection was addressing only one part of the natural history of this confusing and contradictory virus. He resolved there and then never to believe anything he read in textbooks unless it was supported by data.

Rich Whitley presented the results of a randomised controlled trial for the treatment of a brain infection caused by herpes simplex, which was another herpesvirus like CMV and VZV. This disease was called HSV encephalitis and a drug, called vidarabine, inhibited HSV in cell cultures. To determine if it could do the same in patients with severe brain infection caused by this virus, Rich, Charlie and other members of the Collaborative Antiviral Study Group had organised a clinical trial. The disease was rare but, by pooling cases from throughout the USA, they could find enough to work out if the drug had any effect in humans. They needed to know if the drug could alter the natural history of this disease and designed their clinical trial so patients were offered either the drug or a matching placebo which looked the same, but didn't have the active ingredient. The allocation to receive this placebo or the drug was generated randomly by computer.

When the study was complete, the code was broken and revealed that those given the drug had a better clinical outcome than those given placebo. These results were received with acclamation because they were the first example from a randomised controlled trial that an antiviral drug could be developed which had efficacy yet was still safe enough to give to humans.

With the combination of these world-class results, it was not surprising that the site review committee recommended further funding for the Alabama group, so they could continue their quest to understand herpesviruses and bring them under control. The team hoped that a drug would one day be developed against CMV, because Sergio had clearly shown that babies born with high levels of CMV in their urine might benefit from reduction of their viral loads.

Paul enjoyed his time in Alabama, a State which was about the same size as England but which had less than 10% of the population. The result was large areas of uncrowded woodland with lakes and plenty of fresh air. The beaches on the south coast were beautiful, with miles of unspoiled white sand. He returned to London enthused by what he had seen in Alabama. Both seminal papers from Sergio and Rich were published in the *New England Journal of Medicine* in 1977. The results of treating HSV encephalitis were welcomed but, unfortunately, many UK scientists remained sceptical of the observation that natural immunity in women did not always protect their babies against congenital CMV. At scientific meetings, they stated that CMV should follow the precedent set by rubella, citing a statement in a recent UK research paper: *since reactivating women possess pre-existing circulating antibody, intrauterine infection of the fetus does not occur and the baby is born healthy and uninfected.* Paul noted that no evidence was provided to support this assertion, which was true for rubella, but not true for CMV. When he asked speakers at scientific meetings to justify why they were repeating this old statement depite the new information recently published in the *New England Journal of Medicine*, they responded that the discrepancy might represent something unusual about the population in Alabama!

The highest quality of evidence that could be provided about a disease came from the results of a randomised controlled trial. Intermediate quality evidence came from studying groups of patients (cohorts), usually from one centre, whose experience of a condition was used to describe its natural history. The third and lowest quality evidence was summarised as *contemporary medical opinion*. Paul was frustrated by the tendency in the UK to elevate this last category to appear superior to the evidence provided by experimental data in the case of CMV; he thought they were behaving more like revisionist historians than scientists. Nevertheless, he had to ignore this to focus on passing his final Medical School exams, working as a junior doctor and then obtaining a post to train in medical virology. Having done all these things, he applied for a training fellowship to return to the Alabama lab, but for a whole year this time.

When Paul arrived back in Alabama, he was introduced to the other research fellow the lab had accepted for that year; Dr Martha Yow. She was already a Professor at Baylor College of Medicine in Houston and had arranged a fellowship to focus on CMV for a sabbatical year. The contrast between the established Professor from Texas and the young trainee from London, without an established academic post, was striking. They collaborated well, with Martha's experience in caring for babies damaged by CMV complementing Paul's lab knowledge of contemporary virology techniques.

Both research fellows wanted to control paediatric disease caused by CMV and so were delighted to hear new encouraging results from Rich Whitley and the Collaborative Antiviral Study Group. The drug vidarabine, which worked for encephalitis in adults caused by HSV, also worked in babies who had acquired HSV from their mothers at birth. This rare, but devastating, condition was improved in a randomised controlled trial comparing vidarabine with placebo. Although there were side effects, the results showed that an antiviral drug could be given to neonates and opened the way to consider treating babies with CMV if, and when, a suitable drug became available.

In the summer of 1981, as Paul's fellowship was coming to an end, other doctors in the USA wondered if there was a treatment for CMV and started to contact the Alabama lab for advice. It was particularly disappointing to tell them that there was no treatment available for CMV, because it was causing progressive blindness in their patients with an average age of about 30. This was a new presentation of CMV and the doctors in the lab rapidly learnt that the patients were all gay men, mostly living in New York, California or Florida. It was clearly a new disease and these young men, like canaries in a mine, were alerting the population to a new condition which damaged the immune system that normally kept viruses like CMV under control. There was widespread speculation that the mysterious infection which was thought to cause this condition might spread to everyone.

It was five years since the bicentennial had brought many visitors to New York, including those with the novel, but unrecognised, virus HIV. On average, people could slow down its replication for about 10 years before it had damaged the immune system so much that CMV was no longer controlled. But these cases in 1981 were not average; they were the first, had been infected with a larger than average dose of HIV because of their lifestyle and had a shorter incubation period so creating the leading edge of a new epidemic. The principles learned from CMV about how a high viral load causes disease were to be applied to HIV and the principles learned from conducting randomised controlled trials of antiviral drugs active against herpesviruses were to be applied to bring HIV under control. However, it would all take too long to be of help to these first young men, who died of AIDS plus CMV plus other opportunistic infections, just like the cases of chickenpox which killed children with leukaemia. It seemed that herpesviruses frequently delivered the *coup de grace* to patients whose immune systems had been damaged.

A scientific paper from California reported that babies could acquire CMV from blood transfusion. The ones who became sick were those born to seronegative women. Presumably, those born to seropositive women were receiving enough immunity from their mothers to stop them developing illness, even though they became infected from the blood transfusions. This paper was important for two reasons. First, it led to the selection of seronegative donors when blood had to be given to neonates. Second, because the main way mothers transferred immunity to their babies was through antibody passed across the placenta, it implied that vaccines against CMV should aim to stimulate the humoral side of the immune system which was responsible for producing antibody. The possibility that CMV could be transmitted by blood transfusion was also to be broadcast to the world:

Mehmet Ali Agca squinted along the sight of the gun and rotated his body slightly so that an image of his prey appeared at the end of the barrel. He focused intensely and noticed that the man's gold cross around his neck acted as a target for him to aim at. Maintaining his aim, he squeezed the trigger gently.

Mehmet was a troubled man who had practised this on many occasions. Twice before, Mehmet had taken the Browning semi-automatic pistol into the crowds, hoping to be able to shoot the holy man, but to no avail. He would have a third opportunity this Wednesday and was now practising for that possibility.

On the fateful day, 13 May 1981, dawn slowly revealed a clear blue sky over St Peter's Square as Mehmet arrived early to get a good view of the proceedings. One never knew which way the Pope would turn on his perambulations but, one day, he must come within range of Mehmet's gun.

Mehmet's heart skipped a beat, because the Pontiff had turned to come in his direction. There were many more twists and turns on the way which could lead him out of range but, so far, so good.

After another 20 minutes, Mehmet was so excited that he felt in his pocket to slip off the safety catch. Once Pope John Paul II came into range, Mehmet knew he would have only a few seconds to act before someone tackled him, but he had practised well. The moment came; he pulled the gun out of his pocket, squinted down the short barrel, saw the target of the gold crucifix and squeezed the trigger.

The bullet tore out of the barrel at 750 mph. It entered the Pontiff's abdomen and damaged the mesenteric artery, starting serious internal bleeding. By the time the Pope faltered and then was supported by his staff, people in the crowd had wrestled Mehmet to the ground, but not before he had hit the Pope four times.

The Vatican is close to the Agostino Gemelli University Polyclinic, but the transfer of the Pope was impeded by the sheer density of the crowds. The duty surgeon and anaesthetist stood scrubbed ready in theatre to perform their duties, but they had no patient. They were both devout Catholics and prayed that they would not go down in medical history as the doctors who failed to save the Pontiff's life.

They heard the sirens, then the phone rang in theatre to tell them that God's representative on earth was on his way. The anaesthetist checked the four units of blood that were already cross-matched against the Pope's blood group as a matter of routine each time he appeared in public. The anaesthetist ordered another four units of blood just in case and knew that the haematologists would be cross matching it at this very moment.

The doors crashed open as the gurney was driven into theatre at speed. Crossing himself and praying: **forgive me Father***, the anaesthetist gave the syringe full of anaesthetic to the semiconscious Pope and passed an airway into his trachea. Once the Pope was attached to the ventilator, the anaesthetist told the surgeon that he could start.*

Ignoring the niceties of planning to give the patient an aesthetically pleasing scar, the surgeon cut deep and long into the Pontiff's belly. Leaving his assistant to tidy up the wound and to staunch the resulting rather minor bleeding, he dived for the area indicated by the entry wounds of the bullets. The abdomen was full of blood and it was difficult to see what he was doing, even with the suction machine removing the blood as fast as possible.

"Blood-pressure dropping" said the anaesthetist; "I'm giving two units of blood now."

The surgeon kept looking, but could not find the leaking vessel.

"Blood pressure still low; giving units three and four now. Please rush that other blood from the bank and tell them not to bother about cross matching from now on; we're going to need plenty today."

The Pope's heart stopped, as did the surgery. As the last rites were being administered, the doctors successfully defibrillated him with an electric shock. The surgery resumed and the surgeon located the hole in the artery that was pumping blood into the abdomen. He clamped the vessel to stop additional leakage and continued to search for any other sources of bleeding.

"Blood pressure stabilising" said the anaesthetist; "nine units of blood given in total."

The crisis was over, but there was still plenty of work to do to repair the damaged artery and clear up the mess. The surgeon created a colostomy so that the internal wounds to the large bowel could heal. Four more hours later, the Pope's abdomen was closed and he was transferred to the intensive care unit.

It was blood unit number six which contained the stealth virus. Although 60% of blood donors carry this virus somewhere in their body, very few of them transmit through blood transfusion, so the Pope was particularly unlucky. Just as the tension among the doctors and nurses was declining, the stealth virus was making its way around the Pope's body, carried in the white blood cells that accompanied the red blood cells in being suspended in the plasma of the donor blood pack.

The Pope was a senior citizen and so would be expected to require time to recover after major trauma. However, after four weeks, everyone was pleased with his progress and they started to talk about when he could leave hospital. A week later, his personal physician noted a fever. There are many possible reasons for this after major surgery, but the fever was high and spiking so the doctor did not want to take any chances. He arranged for his special patient to have tests which showed that the Pope was having his first infection with the stealth virus.

The stealth virus is normally so mild that most patients are unaware that they have been infected. They usually acquire it when minute amounts of saliva pass from one member of a family to another. Occasionally it can be transmitted during sexual intercourse without causing any symptoms, although this route was obviously not a consideration in the case of the Pope. Instead, he had received a large dose of virus directly into a vein. Because he was part of the 40% of the population who had not acquired it as a child, he did not have any immunity to this virus; his doctors would classify him as seronegative if they had been asked. This combination of a high dose of virus without any prior immunity ensured that the Pope was sick with a high swinging fever. Experts of all nationalities (and religions) were consulted, but only time would help his immune system bring the virus under control. While they waited for this to occur, his doctors performed additional tests and found that the stealth virus had triggered the release of chemical messengers from the body called cytokines. These contributed to his high fever and damaged multiple tissues. The doctors monitored the attack on his kidneys, liver, heart and lungs, giving steroids to try to dampen down the inflammation. This was partially successful, but also suppressed his immune system, helped the stealth virus to replicate and so prolonged the course of his disease. They wanted to give him an antiviral drug to inhibit the stealth virus, but none existed.

Eventually, the immune system got the upper hand and the stealth virus was suppressed to a low level. In time, the colostomy was reversed and the Pope was able to go back to the Vatican, but the invisible stealth virus had kept him in hospital longer than the visible damage caused by the bullet wounds.

Chapter 6:
1982

Although most doctors thought it would never be possible to make antiviral drugs which were safe enough to give to patients in the way that antibiotics were used to control bacterial infections, scientists at the Wellcome Research Laboratories thought otherwise. They had worked for years to synthesise classes of compounds which might interfere with viruses in cell culture, including HSV. Their focus was on a group of naturally occurring compounds called nucleosides, the building blocks which were assembled into polymers to form DNA. One drug was named acycloguanosine because it looked like the natural nucleoside building block of DNA called guanosine, except that the ring structure of the sugar component was broken open so that it no longer formed a circle (hence *acyclo*). This meant that it stopped a virus like HSV from copying its DNA. The drug was very potent and all the clinical trials were reporting that it was safe.

At last, in 1982, the authorities announced that they would give acycloguanosine a licence so that doctors could prescribe it for patients. However, they thought that the name was too unwieldy and decided to call it acyclovir. Thus, the first antiviral drug which was both safe and effective in humans was licensed.

Having shown in 1977 that immune women could deliver babies born with congenital CMV, Sergio's latest paper from Alabama reported that only primary infection in the mother produced babies sufficiently damaged to cause symptoms at birth. An equal number of babies with congenital CMV infection born to seropositive women had no symptoms. This was important, because it showed that maternal immunity offered some protection against disease, although it was not 100% effective at preventing infection. Long term follow up would be required to document how many children suffered ultimately. Sergio acknowledged that some of the cases had been referred to Alabama and that primary infection was easier to diagnose than recurrent infection. Nevertheless, it would take many more years before a population-based study could identify enough cases to define the relative severities of these different types of infection.

The situation was even more complicated than this division of women into two groups, because the seropositives needed to be split, so forming 3 groups of women in total. What we called CMV infection was actually infection with one or more of thousands of different strains, each of which differed very slightly from each other. For example, the DNA of CMV encodes approximately 165 genes each of which produces a protein. One strain might have 164 genes identical to the next strain, but have a mutation in the remaining gene which gave that protein a slightly different function. Some of these altered proteins were the glycoproteins on the surface of the virus which the immune system made antibodies against in order to provide protection against extensive replication. So, a strain of CMV could replicate sufficiently in a pregnant woman to reach the placenta if her natural immune response to a previous strain of CMV did not provide cross protection against the new strain. There was no sight of a lab method which could divide the seropositives into those with reactivation of the virus which had already established itself within their bodies and those with exogenous reinfection which occurred when they encountered another strain of CMV. Just as we needed a fresh flu jab every year to protect against the strains of influenza that were circulating that winter, so we would need a CMV vaccine which covered every strain of CMV.

Later in 1982, a medical school in London, the Royal Free, decided to recruit their first medical virologist. This teaching hospital had performed the first renal transplant in the UK, had an active programme developing bone marrow transplantation and was planning to start liver transplantation. Just like in Seattle, the bone marrow transplant patients were getting major clinical problems with opportunistic infections, especially CMV. Paul reviewed the details of the post and thought it would provide an ideal opportunity to develop laboratory tests for CMV and evaluate them in practice. These evaluations could be performed in material from patients, so meeting his objective of never having to put samples into cell cultures. Paul was appointed to the post, reorganised the lab towards providing rapid diagnosis of viruses of medical importance and focused on developing assays for CMV as his main research objective just as he had planned back in 1976. He thought the main focus would be on transplant patients, but the new epidemic of AIDS occupied an increasing amount of his time.

Billy Rogers had always known he was different from the others at school. He was as happy socialising with the girls as with the boys and did not spend all his time fantasising about naked women; in fact, he was more attracted by glossy photos of handsome men.

When he got a job in Brighton away from the parochial attitudes of his small village in Sussex, his life changed. He felt at home in the active gay scene there and, boy, was it active! He enjoyed the hedonistic lifestyle and looked forward to his evening fun all the time he was at work.

By the time of his 30th birthday, Billy was starting to slow down. He knew that he would grow old one day, but surely 30 was too early? He wondered if he had caught an infection and so went to visit the discrete clinic that had helped him on a couple of previous occasions when he had gonorrhoea. He liked the fact that the staff did not judge his lifestyle, but just gave him the treatment he needed. Although they also gave him condoms and advised about safe sex, they did not moralise at him. He felt sure they would be just as supportive this time, despite the fact that he had never got into the rubber scene.

This time, the doctor was not so sanguine, because the clinical diagnosis was clear:

"Billy, you've picked up AIDS this time. We'll need some blood to check how many CD4 T-cells you have, because that guides us to how far along the disease has progressed. They're a special type of T-lymphocyte that help the immune system fight infections."

"Is there any treatment for this?"

"We assume it's caused by a virus, but don't know its name and there's certainly no treatment for it, but we have treatments for some of the infections you might get down the line."

"So, I need to use condoms from now on to avoid these infections?"

"Billy; it's a bit late for you and condoms. You must be infectious, so you should abstain from sex with other people. If you can't do that, you

should inform them that you have AIDS and use condoms. Our counsellor will help you with some role-play to help you tell any sexual partners about this disease."

Billy was devastated at the thought of his active life coming to an end but, to be honest, felt too tired at the moment anyway. He returned a week later to hear his results:

"Normally, you'd have about 1,000 of these helper CD4 T lymphocytes in each tiny drop of your blood. Your count has dropped by over 90% and now stands at just 75. You're at risk of getting several different infections, so need to go to our specialist clinic in the hospital straight away if you get any problems with your vision, any fever or any spots on your skin."

"Can't I keep coming back here?"

"You can come back here if you want to, but we'll need to send you up to the other specialists because it's likely you'll need to come into hospital from time to time."

Billy was reading about what was on in Brighton when a small shadow moved across the paper. He moved his eyes again and it reappeared, passing slowly across the paper as if it was floating there. The sensation was weird and he could make this thing come and go by moving his eyes from side to side. That doctor had told him to report any problems with his eyes, so he decided to go back to the clinic. He did not want to go to the main hospital for something that seemed so trivial.

"Billy, you may have a serious problem with your eyes. Please go now to this ward and I'll let them know you're on your way."

The doctor put drops in his eyes and stared into them using a bright light.

"You have an infection called the stealth virus which has crossed from your blood into your eyes. Normally, this is prevented by your immune system but, as you know, you have only a few CD4 T-lymphocytes left."

"Is there any treatment?"

"No, I'm afraid there isn't. It's likely to get worse, so I'll ask social services to come round and see how they can help you."

The woman from social services was very matter-of-fact when she came to visit his flat:

"When your doctor tells you it's time, we can move you into some sheltered accommodation where people will be able to help look after you."

Billy went back for regular checkups and was pleased they signed him off work, because he was too fatigued to do anything. The eye thing was his only problem and didn't seem too bad, compared to all the people he had read about who had died in Brighton from AIDS. Two weeks later, his sanguine response was challenged when he suddenly lost most of his vision in one eye. He managed to get to the hospital by keeping the affected eye shut as he walked along slowly, but was shocked at what he was told:

"I'm sorry Billy, but the lining of your right eye, called the retina, has detached. We'll do some minor surgery to try to put it back, but you'll need to wear glasses with a special lens on that side and you may not get much useful vision out of it. It's also time to consider moving to live where people can help you to get around without bumping into things."

Billy was shocked again when the social services woman took him to the hospice. Many of the people there were old, but he was not yet 31. He hated looking at the other people sitting in chairs all day, covered with a blanket. Nature then took its course and wiped out the vision in his other eye so he could not see the old people even if he wanted to.

The stealth virus process that was damaging his eyes was also affecting other parts of his body, including his brain. It was lucky that Billy could not see himself deteriorate as he moved over the next few weeks to resemble the elderly wheelchair-bound patients. He lost all understanding of what was happening to him and lost control of his bowels and bladder as well, before he was mercifully released from this world.

Chapter 7:
1983- 1984

First, one researcher ran up and down the steps of the Philadelphia Museum of Art to get his photograph taken just like the scene in the film *Rocky*, then another researcher took his place. The first CMV international workshop was being held in Philadelphia in April 1983 and they were taking the opportunity to explore the city.

The meeting was organised by Stanley Plotkin, an expert in developing vaccines, who had already helped steer polio vaccines and rubella vaccines through to licensure. He had long been interested in CMV and wanted to see this virus follow the other two in being controlled by vaccination. Stanley opened the meeting by announcing that he had sent a letter on behalf of all attendees to wish Pope John Paul II well, to hope that he was making a speedy recovery from our favourite virus and to ask for an official blessing for the CMV meeting. The telegram providing the blessing arrived the day before the official dinner at the Academy of Music, but when Stanley read it to the audience, most people assumed he was making a joke.

The first workshop was a great success. Anyone in the world who knew anything about CMV was there, but that only amounted to about 200 people. Although the virus caused major problems for pregnant women, neonates, transplant recipients, AIDS patients and now the Pontiff, CMV was ignored by most medical researchers.

Back in London, Paul was looking at the results of a study; the first he had set up since being appointed to the Royal Free. Traditional cell cultures typically took 2-3 weeks to reveal the presence of CMV by producing changes to the shape of the cells. The development of this *cytopathic effect* was characteristic of CMV and had led Tom Weller to give the virus its name. Paul had tried to accelerate the process by using a new approach. He knew that the virus had been taken up into the cells within an hour of the clinical sample being inoculated but, for some reason, these cells took weeks to reveal this; the conventional approach was using *the wrong end point* by waiting for this late event as a means of making a diagnosis. He decided to use a new reagent to identify if the cells contained CMV; a monoclonal antibody.

The development of monoclonal antibodies had just been awarded the *Nobel Prize in Physiology or Medicine* in 1984. Monoclonal antibodies were produced by individual B-lymphocytes and so were pure reagents which worked consistently week by week. In contrast, antisera raised in animals contained multiple antibodies and varied from batch to batch. Paul had obtained a monoclonal antibody specific for CMV and had used it to stain cells in the lab inoculated the day before with clinical samples. The presence of CMV was revealed when the cells were illuminated under the ultraviolet microscope, because the monoclonal antibody had been coupled to an indicator molecule which fluoresced bright green. The results were good enough to replace the older method for testing urine or saliva, because speed was of the essence when telling the bone marrow transplant clinicians which of their patients had active infection with CMV. Unfortunately, it was less able to detect the smaller amounts of CMV found in the blood, so he would need to develop additional tests for this viraemia. Paul played around with several possible names for this new test to help people remember that they should now request it to diagnose CMV infection. He settled on DEAFF, which stood for Detection of Early Antigen Fluorescent Foci, because everyone knew that CMV caused sensorineural deafness, so the pun should remind them that this test was specific for CMV. The results were a significant step forward in rapid diagnosis and were published in the *Lancet*.

The number of patients who had received bone marrow transplants in London was relatively small, but the DEAFF test results looked fairly clear-cut and were the opposite of what Paul was expecting. It was accepted that a seropositive donor of a solid organ could transmit CMV to a recipient, so the same was assumed for bone marrow transplants. However, these results said the opposite; seropositive patients did not do worse and actually did better if the donors of their bone marrow were also seropositive.

Bone marrow transplantation was different, because the organ being transplanted was responsible for mounting immune responses. What if the donors were transmitting immune cells specific for CMV to the recipient rather than virus? Paul wanted to test this possibility directly by giving a CMV vaccine to seronegative donors and seeing if they could transfer some immunity to their sibling when they gave their bone marrow. The problem was, no one had made a CMV vaccine so, instead, they decided to use a vaccine against tetanus.

Nearly 40 patients were selected who were due to donate marrow to their brother or sister. The donors were randomly assigned to not be immunised or to receive a vaccine 7 days before their bone marrow was harvested. After the marrow had engrafted, the patients had more antibody against tetanus in their blood if their sibling donor had been given vaccine. They made even higher levels of antibody if the vaccine was given to both donor and recipient. The antibodies against tetanus would not benefit the patients but, by volunteering for this study, they had shown how CMV vaccines could be evaluated in the future. Once vaccines against CMV became available, they should be given to both donor and recipient about a week before the marrow was harvested from the former and given to the latter. A paper reporting this was published in the *Lancet*.

In Alabama, Bob Pass considered the results in front of him. As a paediatrician, he recognised that children often acquired CMV from their siblings. He wondered if the contemporary arrangements for day care centres to look after the children of working parents had altered the natural history and accelerated acquisition of CMV because young children were now exposed to larger numbers of others at an earlier age. Furthermore, he wanted to investigate whether newly infected children could pass the virus on to their mothers, which could be medically important if they were pregnant.

He had an easy way of broaching these questions because his own children were attending day care. Having explained the background to other parents, he had studied local day care centres to address these possibilities and the results looked fairly clear-cut. Where day care centres had no children excreting CMV in their saliva or urine, there was a very low rate of other children, or parents, acquiring CMV. If a day care centre had at least one child excreting CMV, then transmission was common among children and their parents. The highest risk was found when a child under three had CMV, presumably because they were not trained to deal with their excretions hygienically and so served as a ready source of virus. A major contribution to acquiring CMV during pregnancy could thus be attributed to contact with young children, either one's own, or those that he/she socialised with, especially where many congregated together at places like day care centres. The results had important implications for transmission of this virus, as well as for occupational exposure and were published in the *New England Journal of Medicine.*

Sue Rogers led a busy and fulfilling life. When she and her husband discussed having a family, they realised that they could not afford to pay the mortgage if Sue stopped work. So they planned for her to take only a short period of maternity leave and return to work full-time after the birth of each of the two children they longed for.

Sue conceived early, had a normal pregnancy and an uneventful delivery. She and her husband were delighted to take home their new baby son Tommy and doted on him. Sue loved being a mother and regretted her decision to go back to work as soon as possible, although she knew that, because of the mortgage, she had no option. Sue worked as a secretary and arranged for a local day care centre to look after her son while she went to work. She felt guilty leaving him and longed for the time when she could collect him in the evening because she believed that a good mother should really be looking after him at home at this critical age. To compensate for her guilt driven by financial imperative, she always picked him up, gave him a cuddle and a big kiss before taking him home to the family house she was helping to pay for.

Little Tommy was becoming quite a handful. Sue felt more tired than usual and put it down to looking after the toddler. Once she realised she had missed her period, the penny dropped and she bought a pregnancy test. The blue colour developing in front of her eyes told her that she would be a mother of two small children before the year was out.

Sue collected Tommy as usual and gave him a hug and a kiss. What she did not know is that Tommy had recently acquired stealth virus from other toddlers through playing with toys contaminated with saliva. He was now infectious to others, although he had no symptoms himself. His saliva contained stealth virus and he transmitted it to Sue when she kissed him that evening. After a month, the stealth virus spread quietly in her blood to all parts of her body, including the growing placenta. Sue had not encountered stealth virus as a child and so had no prior immunity to it. In two out of three such seronegative women the stealth virus gets naturally trapped at the placenta and does no harm to the developing baby. However, Sue was the unlucky one woman in three in whom the virus did transmit. She still had no symptoms and so could not ask her doctors to do any tests. It was only when they said that the results of the routine ultrasound tests showed slow growth that she realised things were not quite right.

Sue worried about her baby while she waited for the follow up appointment. When the letter did finally plop through her letterbox she stared at it, wondering what the tests would reveal. Sue had a series of detailed ultrasound examinations which showed that the baby's head, in particular, was growing slowly; more slowly than the rest of the body. She was warned that the baby might have a serious problem, so she was not looking forward to the birth in the way she should have been.

Her labour was easy, because it was a second baby and the head was small. After all the nasty things the doctors had told her about, Sue was relieved to see that her new daughter looked normal, with two arms, two legs and only one head. The doctors did some tests and told Sue that Rachel had stealth virus. They explained that this virus could affect Rachel's development, particularly her brain and hearing.

Having been told this, Sue was anxious when she took Rachel for the appointments with lots of doctors. The neurologist was concerned about the brain damage that his examination revealed. He warned Sue that they would not know for quite a while how this virus would ultimately affect Rachel, because the damage varied between patients and often worsened over time.

The audiologist was wonderful, did lots of tests and reassured Sue that the hearing was normal. However, she did say that stealth virus can damage hearing progressively, so it was important to bring Rachel back for follow-up appointments. She passed her second hearing test, but the audiologist warned that Rachel might not be able to understand the sounds even if they were being transmitted to the correct part of the brain. At the follow up sessions with the neurologist, Rachel failed to meet many of her developmental milestones, showing that stealth virus had damaged her brain profoundly. Rachel also failed the later hearing tests.

When it was time for Sue to go back to work again, the day care centre declined to take Rachel, because they felt they could not cope with her needs. Sue was angry about this, because the doctors had told her that it was probably children at the day care centre who had given the stealth virus to Tommy who had then passed it on to her who had, in turn, given it to Rachel. She had heard of sibling rivalry, but this was an extreme version where her son had transmitted a virus that had done terrible damage to his unborn baby sister.

Because Sue could not obtain childcare support, she could not go back to work as planned. When she came to the end of the maximum time of maternity leave allowed by law, she had to resign and cancelled Tommy's place at the day care centre to save money. Although she enjoyed being at home with her two children and giving Rachel the support she needed, Sue knew that this was not a sustainable long-term position. The anxiety and stress of trying to cope with the financial pressures, together with the daily reminder of the tragedy of their damaged daughter dramatically changed their previously happy home life.

After a further year, she and her husband had no savings left, could not keep up with the mortgage and the bank repossessed their home. Sue's husband could not handle the financial and emotional stress and left, leaving Sue to cope with a lively son and a mentally affected deaf daughter in poor housing while living on social security. She rued the day that stealth virus had come into her life and wondered if the doctors ever added up the full costs that this virus inflicted on people's lives.

Chapter 8: 1984-1986

Stanley Plotkin published his vaccine results in the *Lancet* in 1984. He had taken a strain of CMV in the lab, called Towne, and passed it many times in cell culture. This was a standard way of attenuating a virus to make a vaccine, much as Michiaki Takahashi had done for VZV. Stanley had given the vaccine or a matching placebo to patients awaiting kidney transplant and wanted to see if it would protect them from CMV disease or even CMV infection. The results showed that the vaccine was safe and greatly reduced the severity of CMV disease. However, it did not prevent disease or infection. The results were encouraging for patients who were receiving a substantial CMV challenge in the form of an infected transplanted organ plus potent immunosuppressive drugs. However, they were not as impressive as people had come to expect from live attenuated vaccines, which had dramatically controlled polio, measles, rubella and mumps. Further development of this vaccine was thus slowed down and moved towards people who were not receiving immunosuppressive drugs.

All clinical trials must have controls; that is, patients given a standard treatment whose performance is known. Where no established treatment exists, patients should be randomised to receive placebo or the drug under investigation. But, once a drug has been shown to be superior to placebo, then it becomes the standard against which a new drug should be compared. The field of antiviral therapy had moved on sufficiently that there were now two drugs which could go head to head to determine which was superior in terms of efficacy, safety or both.

Rich Whitley had shown in 1977 that vidarabine was better than placebo for the treatment of HSV encephalitis and so his next study was to compare vidarabine with acyclovir in the same disease. A new cohort of patients with encephalitis caused by HSV was thus recruited and offered randomisation to vidarabine or to acyclovir. The study was completed in 1986 and showed that acyclovir was superior to the older drug, both for efficacy and safety. Thus, acyclovir became the new gold standard treatment for this serious disease. As befits a landmark study, the first to compare one antiviral drug with another, the scientific paper was published in the *New England Journal of Medicine.*

By 1986, the use of MMR vaccine to control measles, mumps and rubella infection in childhood had reduced the number of cases of congenital rubella in the USA down to very low levels by decreasing the chance that pregnant women would encounter a child with rubella. In contrast, the UK had followed a policy of immunising women of childbearing age but allowing rubella to circulate in children. In theory, this should have protected unborn babies from rubella but, in practice, there were too many ways for women to miss out on getting the vaccine before they became pregnant. In the UK, cases of congenital rubella stayed stubbornly high and were being controlled by selective termination of pregnancy when women with rashes were diagnosed with rubella. The UK authorities decided to copy the USA experience by swapping policies to give MMR vaccine to all children. This rapidly interrupted transmission of rubella in the community and cases of congenital rubella promptly disappeared. Thus, in this case, the controls were not randomised within a study, but came from comparisons between two countries. The principle was established that immunising children was an effective and efficient way of protecting their mothers and their unborn siblings. It was also an effective way of protecting adults in general who might suffer from infections acquired from children.

James Gordon was looking forward to being useful once again. After he retired from his post as manager of a local bank branch, he enjoyed socialising with people at the golf club. Neither he nor his wife were very good at golf, but they were both fair bridge players and spent many a happy afternoon in the clubhouse demonstrating their skills. But when his wife died suddenly, James' whole world fell apart. The neighbours were supportive, but he did not want to go to places that he and his wife had frequented in the past, because they stimulated too many memories. So, when his daughter suggested that he might like to buy a house near to them and help look after his grandchildren, he jumped at the chance.

Old habits die hard and the bank manager that still lived within his body was delighted to see how cheap property was in Leicestershire compared with Surrey. He sold his house, bought a three-bedroom detached house with manageable garden and still had £100,000 left over. He put this into a long-term bond with his old bank and looked forward to monitoring the accumulating interest.

He had enjoyed playing games and reading stories to his own children and rapidly got into the same routine with his two young grandchildren. He drove to his daughter's house every morning and took the children the short distance to school, so freeing her up to get to work without time pressures. In the evenings, he collected the children from school and gave them a quick snack while they waited for their mum to come home. He then took his leave, because he did not want to overstay his welcome and interfere when his son-in-law came home. Although they all got on well, he was sufficiently worldly wise to understand that everyone needs their own personal time and space. This double dose of seeing his grandchildren every day was just the right amount of human contact and responsibility for James, because he was content to settle into the routine of reading The Times *every morning, having a lunchtime snooze and watching the evening news before retiring early to fall asleep listening to* Radio *4.*

He doted on his grandchildren and made sure he gave them each a kiss at the school gates. That was when the stealth virus got him. James had led a sheltered life, having married his childhood sweetheart who was the only girl he had ever kissed. His exposure to saliva had thus been minimal (unless one included the requirement early in his training with the bank to seal letters to customers with his own spittle). He had therefore reached 71 years of age without encountering stealth virus and so was seronegative. Two months after moving house he woke with a fever and felt lethargic. He struggled to get out of bed (after all, his new role in life was really important), showered and managed to reach his daughter's house. She took one look at his pale, sweaty face, felt his rapid pulse, thought he was having a heart attack and called for an ambulance. Her diagnosis was incorrect, but she meant well. The doctors told her that he did have some heart disease but that it was not the cause of his current illness. Instead, they told her that he had **a virus** *and did some blood tests. That was when the stealth virus was discovered.*

It took him three months to recover from the episode of primary infection, but he never went back to being his old self. The shock of the fever, the toxicity of the cytokines, the trauma of the hospital admission and the third disruption to his way of life within a year all took their toll. Although he was now better physically, his daughter was concerned to see how much he had aged mentally in such a short time. He was forgetful and disorientated, so she wondered if it was safe to have him looking after the children. During this time, his daughter had coped with the childcare duties. By the time he was declared fit enough to drive again, the children were a little older and it was decided that they were responsible enough to walk to school together. Thus, James' new role in life did not work out exactly as planned. As the grandchildren grew up, he felt excluded from their childhood. He began to rue the day that he had moved to Leicestershire and could not quite remember why he had decided to do so. He also forgot about that bond from his bank that he had previously looked forward to monitoring.

His daughter was shocked at how rapidly he developed dementia, yet it was the stealth virus that had accelerated his decline and interfered with the plans of his extended family. He became a new dependent for her to look after, rather than the contributor to her family's quality of life that she had anticipated. In her limited spare time, she wondered why the doctors did not screen new grandparents to make sure they were immune to viruses carried by children and give them vaccines if necessary to protect their retirement years. If they couldn't do that, why didn't they give a vaccine to all children so that grandparents would be protected indirectly?

Chapter 9: 1987-1988

In Boston, David Snydman got the results of his double-blind, randomised, placebo-controlled trial of immunoglobulin in seronegative renal transplant patients whose organ donors were seropositive. He had prepared immunoglobulin from seropositive blood donors and given it to half of the renal patients in a randomised fashion. The results showed a significantly reduced number of cases of severe CMV disease, but no effect on CMV infection. The results clearly implied that antibody made during natural infection had an effect on CMV transmitted from the donor. The results were published in the *New England Journal of Medicine*, but people had difficulty believing them:

"How can immunoglobulin have an effect on CMV disease when it doesn't have an effect on the infection which causes that disease?"

They were clearly unaware of the 1975 paper from Alabama, reporting that a high viral load was associated with disease, so that reducing the quantity of virus could plausibly reduce disease without necessarily abolishing infection.

The scientist who developed acyclovir, called Trudy Elion, was awarded the *Nobel Prize for Physiology or Medicine* in 1988 for this discovery; one of only nine women at that time who had become a Nobelist. Her lab also had a related compound called ganciclovir which had activity against CMV but was predicted to have important side-effects because it was toxic to cultures of bone marrow. The drug was developed by a different pharmaceutical company, but without conducting placebo-controlled trials. Instead, AIDS patients with early CMV retinitis were recruited and randomised to receive ganciclovir immediately or only when their retinitis progressed. The results showed that the toxicity from giving ganciclovir early was justified, because it protected the vision of these seriously ill patients who only had months to live. Ganciclovir was licensed on this basis but, once the drug was available for AIDS patients, it could be prescribed for additional individual patients at the discretion of their doctor.

The next study from London produced interesting results. It seemed likely that patients with natural immunity against CMV were not completely protected against getting a new strain of virus if they received an organ from an infected donor. The problem was how to prove this? There were thousands of different strains of CMV, so a study would need carefully chosen controls. Paul decided to take advantage of an *experiment of medicine*; that is, to investigate in detail the cases of patients selected because they could be particularly informative.

When donors die, multiple organs become available for transplantation. Paul decided to collect examples where organs from a single donor had been transplanted into more than one recipient at the Royal Free. By collecting CMVs from each of the recipients and typing them, they could prove that a particular strain had infected more than one patient if the two patients had the same type of CMV. If one recipient lacked antibodies against CMV but the other had been seropositive before transplant, this would prove that CMV in the donated organ had reinfected the latter patient. The team collected a series of such examples, proved that reinfection occurred and, importantly, showed that the severity of CMV disease was less than that of primary infection but greater than that of reactivation. In fact, when seropositive patients received organs from uninfected donors, they frequently reactivated CMV that usually did not produce any symptoms. These results were important for understanding the natural history of CMV and had direct implications for attempting to control this infection by means of vaccination and so the paper was published in the *Lancet.*

In 1988, *Science* published a remarkable paper by Kary Mullis who would go on to receive the *Nobel Prize for Chemistry* five years later for this invention.

Mullis was a nonconformist, out-of-the-box original thinker who described how he had gained the insight which led to his discovery. Late at night, he was driving up into the Californian hills when his girlfriend fell asleep beside him. To keep himself awake, he reviewed the experiment he had been conducting in the lab that day. DNA polymerase enzymes (like the one HSV uses to replicate which is poisoned by acyclovir) take one strand of DNA and copy it, so that a double stranded DNA molecule is formed. However, they need a small stretch which is partially double stranded to latch onto before they can move along the single stranded part (the template) copying the

DNA as they go. Mullis had learned that he could command the enzyme where to bind simply by adding single stranded DNA primers which bound to different parts of the molecule. Of course, once the enzyme reached the end of the template it would stop, so that the ends of the molecules would always be the same, irrespective of where the enzyme started from.

He then wondered what would happen if he heated the new double stranded DNA to separate it into two single stranded molecules and added the primer again. He could be sure that the enzyme would latch on to the double stranded portion and keep going until it reached the other end of the molecule. By then, he would have doubled the amount of DNA that he had started with.

The flash of inspiration came when he realised he could do both parts at once. A pair of primers, staggered so that they bound different parts of the single stranded DNA, could direct the polymerase to double the amount of the input molecule. If he then repeated the process, he would have four times as much as he had started with, then eight times then 16 times etc. Mullis says that he realised the technique was so elegant and so simple that he knew that evening it would win him the Nobel Prize. He decided to call the technique PCR, for polymerase chain reaction.

There was just one fly in the ointment of his elegant scheme. Each time he heated the chemicals he destroyed the enzyme so, after each cycle, he had to open the container and add more enzyme. This did not bother Mullis, because he was an ideas man, not a pragmatist. He got a technician to do the laborious work to prove his point.

The article in *Science* was influential and Paul's lab in London decided to see if it could be made into a practical way of detecting and quantifying CMV in clinical samples, particularly in blood, where the DEAFF test was not sensitive enough. By using the DNA from CMV as the template, they hoped to produce a rapid and sensitive test for CMV in the blood of patients.

Kate Peters had been bothered by urinary tract infections since she was a little girl. Each one of these had been treated with antibiotics, but each infection damaged part of her kidneys so, by the time she was 18, she had very little function left and had to receive kidney dialysis three times a week.

Kate was a brave girl who bore her disease with good cheer, but her parents were distressed to see how tired she was becoming and how much of her young life was spent attached to a machine. When they heard from her doctors that a transplant was the best way of managing the disease, her father immediately volunteered to be the donor. He had lots of investigations to make sure his kidney would be compatible with Kate's. These included blood tests to ensure he was not infected with viruses which could be transmitted with the organ, such as HIV or hepatitis B. Eventually, he got the all-clear and the doctors gave them a date for the transplant.

There was a great sense of anticipation in the Peters family as the day approached when dad and daughter would both go into hospital together. Kate was very grateful to her father for volunteering and he felt good about his altruism. The surgery was technically flawless and the new kidney functioned immediately. Kate's general health improved within days as she obtained better renal function courtesy of her father.

Unbeknown to both of them, Kate also acquired stealth virus from her father's kidney. She was one of the 40% without immunity whereas he was one of the 60% who had acquired the virus in the past. Kate had only been home for 10 days when the sudden onset of a high fever required her to be readmitted to hospital. She then developed another problem because the stealth virus triggered her immune system to release cytokines and reject the kidney. This responded to immunosuppressive drugs, but these in turn encouraged the stealth virus to replicate, so setting up a vicious circle. By the time the infection and the rejection had both been brought under control, her transplanted kidney had such poor function that she needed to return to dialysis.

Like he had done before, Kate's father watched her attached to the dialysis machine three times a week. Only this time was different, for he had a scar on his flank and only one functioning kidney himself.

Kate's mother had initially been reluctant to donate a kidney and was content to let her husband demonstrate his bravery. Yet, he clearly could not donate his last remaining kidney, so she would have to consider donating one of hers. She had observed how well he had withstood the surgery, yet knew that he was stronger, braver and more robust than her. She wondered if the investigations would show that her kidney was not compatible with Kate's so that she could appear to be brave without actually having to go through with it.

In the event, the transplant doctor told her that all the blood tests were fine and she was not infected with HIV or hepatitis B. She asked the doctor if Kate might have the same problem with stealth virus again if she was transplanted with her mother's kidney. He told the mother that, like her husband, she was one of the 60% of the population who carried the stealth virus, but that, if infection was transmitted to her daughter, it should be much milder this time because Kate's immune system was ready to fight the virus.

"Think of it as if she's had a vaccine" said the doctor. "Kate had a stormy time, but now is at least immune to this stealth virus."

"Why then can't you make a real vaccine to give to everyone who needs a transplant?"

The doctor smiled at the naïve question; it was easy to forget how little medical and scientific knowledge the average person had!

"I'm afraid there's no possibility of that. Vaccines work by inducing immune responses and the stealth virus is notorious for evading immunity. It would be impossible to make a vaccine."

"Why can't you screen donors to find out who has this virus?"

"We do, which is how I can tell you that you have had this infection in the past. But we can't use that information to halt a planned transplant, because we would have to cancel 60% of them. Would you like me to tell you today that you can't be a donor so that your daughter will have to remain on dialysis?"

If she was truthful to herself, the mother did not want to lose her kidney and did not want to go through the trauma of a major operation. Yet, she could not deny this chance of a normal life to her daughter and would forever feel like a coward if she failed to follow the bravery of her husband. Thus, trying to hide her real feelings, she volunteered to donate.

This time it was mother and daughter who went to the hospital together and it was the father who had to wait. The surgery was uneventful and the kidney functioned well. The doctors monitored Kate closely for stealth virus using DEAFF test, but her primed immune system worked so well that the virus only appeared once in her urine and disappeared immediately when they gave her the new antiviral drug called ganciclovir, which had just been licensed, before the virus had a chance to trigger those noxious cytokines. The parents were concerned to hear that stealth virus had come back into their life again, but the doctors were reassuring. They explained that the virus may have reactivated from Kate or she may have been reinfected with virus from her mother's kidney. Both of these were much milder than the primary infection she had acquired from her father's kidney in the past. The fact that the virus in the urine had responded to the new treatment was a good sign.

Kate returned home and never had to go back onto dialysis. She looked so healthy and happy that her mother was pleased she had found the courage to donate. However, every time she saw her husband's scar, she could not help feeling that he had lost a kidney in order to vaccinate his daughter against stealth virus.

Chapter 10:
1989-1993

Bob Rubin was a larger-than-life infectious diseases physician with an encyclopaedic experience of managing opportunistic infections in the immunocompromised host as part of his clinical practice in Boston. He had just been asked to write an editorial to accompany a scientific paper which would shortly be published in a medical journal. A group of heart transplant clinicians had noticed that their patients who developed CMV disease also tended to get other problems, including graft rejection and accelerated atherosclerosis in the newly transplanted heart. Bob called his editorial *the indirect effects of cytomegalovirus infection on the outcome of organ transplantation*, to emphasise that active infection with this virus may trigger adverse events which were not unique to CMV. In this way, CMV could damage patients without necessarily declaring itself clinically. Nobody would realise that CMV was making this contribution to overall outcome unless they were looking for it specifically. In contrast, the *direct effects* of CMV were the end organ diseases caused when the virus disseminated in the bloodstream to reach organs like the lungs or retina. These diseases could be identified in individual patients when the typical inclusion bodies were seen in biopsies or in autopsies.

In London, Paul was delighted to receive the statistical analysis of the new study his research group had conducted. CMV disease, particularly affecting the eyes, had clearly become a major problem for AIDS patients starting with the first cases which had presented while he was still in Alabama. He thought that there could also be another way in which CMV was causing damage to AIDS patients, much as transplant patients developed *indirect effects*. CMV could be interacting with HIV to accelerate the rate at which that virus caused AIDS. There were multiple ways in which the two viruses could interact, including the fact that both viruses damage the immune system, but his attempts to raise grant money to study them had all been rejected. It was also difficult to find appropriate controls, because almost all gay men with AIDS were seropositive.

He decided to study haemophiliacs, who had acquired HIV through infusion of contaminated blood products. The Royal Free had the largest cohort of patients with haemophilia in Europe and had stored serum samples going back before HIV appeared. This meant that the researchers could establish the time when most people had acquired HIV and so ask if those with CMV on board developed AIDS more quickly. About 60% of the haemophiliacs were CMV seropositive, leaving 40% to act as the control group. The bad news was that his grant request to investigate active CMV infection in urine had been turned down, so they only had serum available. They could measure antibodies to determine which patients were CMV seropositive, but this was only a rough guide to who was at risk of active infection with CMV. Nevertheless, without grant support it was all they could do.

The results showed that significantly more haemophiliacs developed AIDS if they were also CMV seropositive. It was the first report that CMV could interact with HIV in humans and was published in the *Lancet.* Paul thought this was similar to the way another herpesvirus, Epstein-Barr virus or EBV, interacted with malaria to cause Burkitt's lymphoma. This tumour was caused by EBV but was found only in children living below a certain altitude in Africa or New Guinea. The children who developed the disease were those who got malaria at the same time as EBV, because malaria, like EBV, stimulated B-lymphocytes to form the B-cell tumour. Most children high up in the mountains got EBV infection, but were protected against the tumour, because the mosquitoes could not fly high enough to give them the malaria cofactor. Given this precedent, Paul decided to use the term *cofactor* to describe the relationship between HIV and CMV, but this term and the concept were controversial and it is fair to say that most people did not believe the results. The *Lancet* paper proposed that a placebo-controlled trial of a drug active against CMV should be conducted to address the possible cofactor relationship, but most investigators were hostile to this suggestion, because the only drug licensed for CMV, ganciclovir, gave side-effects and so might do more harm than good.

The sun was reflecting off the waves of the Pacific Ocean as another beautiful dawn broke over San Diego in March 1989. Six years had elapsed since the first international CMV workshop and the diehard group of researchers interested in this virus had gladly responded to the invitation from the husband-and-wife team of Debbie and Steve Spector to travel to California for the second.

The CMV researchers could immediately see the implications of the cofactor hypothesis when the results were presented and discussed, but the problem lay with the community of HIV researchers who were too focused on providing care for AIDS patients to consider the complexities of how another virus might be hastening the demise of their patients. The CMV meeting was very successful and the group committed to meeting every two years from now on.

Bob Rubin's ability to capture the zeitgeist came to the fore again. He had been asked to write an editorial to accompany a paper in the *New England Journal of Medicine*. CMV pneumonitis was the most feared form of CMV disease and most cases occurred after bone marrow transplantation, as we saw with Julie Jefferies. It was suspected that CMV infection of the lung occurred soon after transplant but that, once the new marrow engrafted, lymphocytes from the donor mounted inflammatory reactions to attack the virus, thereby damaging the lungs in the process. Clinicians had passed a small tube into the lungs soon after transplant, identified those patients with active CMV infection using the DEAFF test and randomised them to receive treatment with ganciclovir or no treatment. This was a difficult study, because the procedure for sampling the lungs was invasive and ganciclovir was toxic to the newly engrafted marrow. Nevertheless, the results showed that early treatment reduced the important outcomes of CMV pneumonia or death.

Sitting at home in the evening, Bob wondered how to explain what the doctors had done. The TV was on in the background and CNN suddenly announced that the anticipated attack on Baghdad had begun as part of Operation Desert Storm. The announcer explained that the first wave of bombs and missiles would attack the Iraqi air defence radar system in a pre-emptive strike. Eureka! Bob entitled his editorial *preemptive therapy in immunocompromised hosts* and explained how the virus was being tackled before it could cause any harm. Although the approach of sampling the lungs was soon to be replaced by the less invasive approach of monitoring patients for virus in the blood (viraemia), the term preemptive therapy stuck and was used to describe the policy of seeking viraemia or infection in the lungs of transplant patients and treating them before CMV could trigger extensive damage.

Bologna has the oldest university in Europe. Two years had come round quickly as the CMV aficionados congregated there in June 1991 for the third international workshop. Within sight of the tower which leaned as precariously as its more famous namesake in Pisa, they shared delicious pasta dishes with their hosts after discussing at length the virus that preoccupied their working lives.

Karen Fowler was an epidemiologist based in Alabama who was committed to help control deafness caused by CMV. She published the latest natural history study in the *New England Journal of Medicine* showing that primary infection in the mother represented more of a threat to the fetus than did infection of seropositive women. Follow up of a large number of children showed that congenital infection caused disease in both groups, but that the proportion of children with symptoms, and the severity of those symptoms, was increased when women entered pregnancy without antibodies to CMV. As well as providing important information on which to counsel women, these results provided the rationale for attempting to immunise seronegative women as a way of controlling congenital infection.

The person invited to write the accompanying editorial was Martha Yow. To provide perspective, she cited the 1971 review by Tom Weller and concluded that, using his figures, 170,000 children in the USA had developed deafness and neurological impairment since his article had been published by the *New England Journal of Medicine*. Entitling her editorial: *congenital cytomegalovirus disease- 20 years is long enough*, she made an impassioned plea for the development of a vaccine against CMV with the final line: ***we should not wait another 20 years, while thousands of additional children are born seriously handicapped.***

In the same year that Kary Mullis received the Nobel Prize, the London lab showed that PCR could be used for routine diagnosis of CMV. Vince Emery in Paul's lab obtained results which showed that the method for quantifying the PCR results could be made to work so that they would know which patients had a high viral load. Unfortunately, the quantitative method was too cumbersome to use routinely, but there was a way to identify patients at risk of developing high viral loads. The results of a clinical study showed that finding CMV DNA by PCR in two consecutive weekly samples identified patients who were likely to develop a high viral load. Thus, a PCR screening test could be performed to identify patients who should be offered preemptive therapy. CMV could now be detected before it made people ill, so providing an opportunity to treat the infection and prevent disease.

Although these results in transplant patients were encouraging, the same lab got both negative and positive results from two studies in AIDS patients. First, Paul had identified an investigator in the USA who had blood samples stored from haemophiliacs. They tested them for CMV antibodies but failed to reproduce the results of the earlier study which had identified CMV as a cofactor, accelerating the development of AIDS. Paul suspected this was because the measurement of antibody gave only a rough indication of which patients were at risk of active CMV infection and rued the time his grant proposing a study of active CMV infection in the urine had been turned down. Nevertheless, a central feature of research is for results to be confirmed in an independent study so the use of antibody measurements in haemophiliacs had just failed that test. Second, Paul and a research fellow had attended a series of autopsies of AIDS patients and collected samples from multiple organs. They found that most patients had CMV in at least one organ. Clearly, AIDS patients were dying with CMV, but were they dying from it?

Stephen Williams was only 15 and he loved playing the guitar. He spent his school days thinking about what he would do in the evenings with his three like-minded friends who played music as much as possible. They learned chords and practised famous pieces of rock music. As their skills improved, they started to play at birthday parties and then, as they got older, at pubs in the evenings. They did not make much money, but it was enough to maintain their musical instruments and buy beer. They left school as soon as possible and, living with their parents, eked out a nomadic existence moving from one pub to another plus occasional small gigs at the weekends.

The transition came when they started to write their own music and lyrics. They were not bad and kept practising so that they could play well and did so at every opportunity. Their style was rock initially and then progressed to heavy rock, so they decided to change their names and clothing. The jeans and T-shirts were replaced with punk style clothing and Stephen Williams transformed into Stevie Headbanger. They played in this new guise for several weeks and were well received by their young audiences. Then, one evening, a man about the age of Stevie's father approached them after a gig:

"That was pretty good guys; do you have an agent to represent you?"

Within a month, Stevie Headbanger and friends were whisked into a tornado of activity as the agent arranged for them to play at larger venues throughout the country. He provided a minivan and a driver to transport their kit up and down the motorways of the UK. He gave them money to spend and told them that they were doing really well. The travel and playing schedules were hectic so Stevie and the others needed to take naps in the minivan to cope. They were sleeping in a series of bed-and-breakfast places for one night at a time and were becoming exhausted.

Stevie, like many of his musical heroes, experimented with weed, ecstasy and cocaine. But it was not until his band was rehearsing for a gig supporting a nationally acclaimed punk band that he had his first experience with heroin.

"You look knackered mate. You need a pick me up."

The lead guitarist showed Stevie how he survived tours. He found a vein and injected a dose of heroin. Immediately, his eyes sparkled, his fatigue disappeared and he was endowed with energy and enthusiasm.

"It's good for your music too. You'll create loads of new stuff while you're high."

That was the clincher for Stevie, because music was the most important thing in his life. He picked up the same syringe and copied exactly what the older guitarist had done. The sensation hit him instantly. He played like a wild man that evening and got rave responses from the audience, his manager and from the other members of his group. From that moment on, he was a convert to the benefits of heroin. From that moment too, he had converted to HIV-positive, but did not know this yet.

The career of Stevie Headbanger went from strength to strength as the group travelled to venues in Europe as well as in the UK. But the hectic travel schedule, the disrupted sleep cycles plus, for Stevie, his underlying HIV, started to take their toll. The heroin gave him less and less of a boost each time and the manager, in fear of losing a lucrative investment, arranged for Stevie to see a doctor who looked after many pop stars.

"He's one of the best and is very discreet, so you can tell him anything."

The manager dropped him in Harley Street where Stevie looked with trepidation at the imposing Georgian terrace with brass plate on the door. The confidential history of his lifestyle plus blood tests revealed HIV as a major contributor to his fatigue. The doctor started him on two antiviral drugs, told him to abstain from heroin and alcohol and to return in a week.

That week was really strange. Stevie did exactly as the doctor had told him, because he was frightened by the announcement that he had HIV. He knew how many people in the music business had died of AIDS and did not want to follow them. He thought he would miss the boost given by the heroin although, in fact, he had been receiving less benefit from each dose than he had in the past. By abstaining from alcohol he also removed another depressant from his system. The net effect was that he managed to survive the first week and kept up with the reduced number of gigs that the manager arranged. One week later, he got some good news from the doctor in Harley Street:

"You only need to remember two numbers. One thousand is the number of white blood cells of a special type, called CD4 T-lymphocytes or helper T cells that are normally found in healthy people. These

are important because, as the name suggests, they help your body make immune responses to protect you against multiple infections. HIV kills these cells, so that the number in the blood goes down. The second number to remember is one hundred. If we treat your HIV with two antiviral drugs to keep your CD4 count above 100 you should not suffer from any life-threatening infections. You may still develop some other problems which we can talk about later, but keeping the count above 100 is important, so you need to take the medicines regularly and keep coming back for blood tests. The diagnosis of HIV is no longer a death sentence."

"Thanks; I think I can follow that. So, what's my count of these helper cells?"

"When you came to see me last week your count was down to 200, but you've made a good response to treatment and it's already gone up to 215. Keep taking the tablets, avoid heroin and alcohol and your count will increase much further over time. It won't go back to normal, but I can usually keep people like you out of major trouble as long as you follow my advice to the letter. Also, avoid new sexual partners, because they can give you infections which can be serious in their own right, but which also can upset the balance of HIV. Sorry to be a killjoy, but my message is: stick to rock 'n' roll but avoid the drugs and sex."

Stevie left Harley Street determined to follow this advice carefully, because he wanted to stay healthy to play for his audiences. He would not have difficulty avoiding sex, because Stephen Williams had never had a regular girlfriend and Stevie Headbanger was too focused on his music to be interested in women.

Over the next six months, Stevie's CD4 count increased slowly but surely to settle into a new value of 350. The doctor reminded him that this was not normal, but should be enough to stop him dying from major infections. The doctor also told him that his HIV viral load, the amount of virus in his blood, had gone down to a low level, which meant that he was probably not infectious to other people. During this time, Stevie's music had become more mellow, less driven by peaks of heroin or alcohol driven troughs of despair. His audiences, his manager and now his record-

ing company were delighted with the new songs that Stevie and the group were producing. His schedule became less hectic, because the manager could choose well-paid prestigious gigs at a small number of international venues. This gave the band time to be more creative and more time to record their music. It also gave Stevie time to reflect on his life.

Stephen had been born into the poor working class Williams family. His father worked in a factory and told his son that he should do the same. Stevie had now earned more money than his father had in his whole life. He did not understand the investments and tax breaks his manager told him about, but knew that he had already earned enough to buy his parents a new house. Not a council flat mind, a real four bedroomed house standing on its own plot of land with a garden and no noisy neighbours to be heard through a party wall. Stevie realised that he had been stupid sharing that needle, getting addicted to heroin and acquiring HIV. Yet, that doctor had treated him well and given him a second chance. He now felt much better, was less angry with life and more in control of himself. He rather envied his parents living in a new house and wondered if he should buy himself a place when the next block of royalty money came through. What type of house to buy? He did not fancy a flat, because it was too much like his earlier life in that council flat. No, he wanted a house with a garden, but who could he ask to share with him? It was then that his 25-year-old loins reminded him of another part of life that he was neglecting.

Stevie had been to the office of his record company on several occasions, but was now struck by a blonde girl he had not noticed before. She looked beautiful and he kept thinking of her all through the boring contract discussions. Stevie was feeling healthy now his HIV was under control; he was feeling in charge of his life and wanted someone to share his new house with him. He resolved to take action immediately. He had no experience of chatting up girls, because they usually threw themselves at him, but he did have one advantage; he was now a well-known pop star.

"Hello," said Stevie. "I'm Stevie Headbanger."

"Oh, I know who you are Mr Headbanger" Emma replied with a smile.

Nobody had ever called him that before and he smiled back at her.

"I wonder if you'd like to come out for a drink with me one evening?"

"I'd love to" she said. "Which evening did you have in mind?"

"How about Wednesday?"

"Wednesday it is. Where shall we meet?"

"Give me your address and I'll send a car to take you to the cocktail lounge at the top of the Hilton tower. I've been there before and it has a wicked view."

She smiled back:

"That won't be necessary. I've lived all my life in London and can find my way to the Hilton. What time shall we meet?"

"7:30?" he suggested.

"Okay, I'll see you then in the cocktail lounge and thanks for inviting me."

As he descended in the lift, his stomach had a fluttering sensation, but it was due to love not gravity.

Stevie got to the Hilton early, having pulled rank to book a table by the window. Emma looked stunning as she walked into the lounge wearing an electric blue cocktail dress. She chose one of the unfamiliar cocktails and they began to chat. After two cocktails each, he enquired if she was hungry and they adjourned to the restaurant. They just chatted naturally and time flew.

"Stevie, this has been a wonderful evening, but I need to get home now, because my dad doesn't like me being out late and I have to be at work by nine tomorrow morning."

"Can I put you in a taxi?"

"That would be wonderful at this time of night and get me home before Cinderella turns into a pumpkin."

At the end of their second date, Emma let Stevie kiss her on the cheek as she got into the taxi. On their third date, they held hands in the cocktail lounge and had a long passionate kiss at the taxi rank.

"Stevie; I like you very much, but I'm not one of those girls who jump into bed with pop stars."

"Good, because I'm not a pop star who does that sort of thing."

"Would you like me to come to your place to cook you a meal? I'm quite a good chef and I see your schedule's free on Wednesday."

She wore the electric blue cocktail dress again and he longed for her. After the meal and wine they adjourned to the sofa.

"Stevie, please be gentle with me, because I've never done this before, but I think I'm falling in love with you."

"Since we're sharing secrets, I love you too."

She may not have done it before, but her young body was ready. Unfortunately, as a toddler, Emma had acquired stealth virus which had spread in her bloodstream to all parts of her body. At this moment, her salivary glands were producing this unwanted component. Stevie had also acquired stealth virus as a child, but the immune system could not prevent reinfections with the stealth virus. Stevie's reinfection did not produce any symptoms, because the helper CD4 T cells did their job and limited the viral load of the stealth virus. However, in the special case of someone who was HIV positive, stealth virus could stimulate these CD4 cells to produce HIV. This had two effects. First, it competed with the antiviral drugs to drive the replication of Stevie's HIV so that he progressed more rapidly towards AIDS; second, his increased HIV viral load meant that he was more likely to infect a sexual partner. His doctor had told Stevie that he was very unlikely to be infectious; however, the doctor did not know about the reinfection with stealth virus.

As Emma enjoyed the sensation of their lovemaking, her salivary glands released stealth virus to reinfect Stevie. This activated his HIV so that, when they did it again the following week, Stevie gave HIV to Emma. Thus it was that two people shared two viruses that were notorious for being sexually transmitted without either of them having originally been acquired sexually.

The acquisition of stealth virus gave Stevie two further long-term problems. First, by driving the replication of HIV in the presence of the antiviral drugs he was taking, the stealth virus helped to create resistant strains of HIV. The doctors identified the resistant virus when his CD4 count fell and blamed progression of the disease on HIV resistance. They were unaware of stealth virus and even accused Stevie of failing to take the drugs regularly. Second, the stealth virus increased the number of CD8 lymphocytes in his blood as the immune system diverted its resources towards attacking stealth virus rather than keeping HIV under control. If he had lived for three more years he would have benefited from new anti-viral drugs, given in a cocktail of 3, which dramatically controlled HIV replication. But, together with his other problems, stealth virus would send him to an early grave leaving behind a beautiful young widow who was HIV positive.

Chapter 11:
1994-1996

The Eiffel Tower was the icon that the CMV researchers got photographed against as the 4th international workshop met in April 1993 in the *City of Light.* One session was devoted to discussing the precise criteria which should be used to define CMV infection and CMV disease; two terms which were used vaguely. Consensus was reached and the criteria were published to help make different studies more comparable from now on by using agreed endpoints. *CMV infection* was defined as the detection of the virus in any part of the body of a patient. *CMV end organ disease* required CMV infection to be present together with symptoms, plus detection of inclusion bodies in a biopsy taken from the affected organ (except for retinitis, where the typical picture at the back of the eye was accepted to be diagnostic). *CMV syndrome* was to be kept distinct from CMV end organ disease, which was synonymous with Bob Rubin's direct effects. The *indirect effects* of CMV could only be proven in populations of patients, not in individuals.

Back in Alabama, Sergio recognised that several features of contemporary life were interacting to alter the risks of a woman acquiring primary CMV infection during pregnancy. If a seropositive woman breastfed her daughter, there was a good chance that she would give her CMV infection which would not cause any damage provided she had not been denied maternal antibody by being born prematurely. This perinatal infection from breast milk would give her some protection when she grew up to have babies of her own. The daughter might still have a baby born with congenital CMV, but it would be less likely to suffer disease than if she remained seronegative until she became pregnant and then caught primary infection. In this way, breastfeeding could be thought of as a way of immunising females against the risk that the worst ravages of this infection might visit them at a vulnerable time in the future. This pattern of almost 100% of young children acquiring CMV had been universal throughout the globe until the 20th century and was still found in poorer sections of communities in developed countries, but not those in the middle classes who now frequently entered the childbearing years without antibodies against CMV.

However, there were also ways in which breastfeeding could increase the risk of disease. If a seropositive woman breastfed her baby and let her or him mingle with other babies, then they would be a source of virus for other babies and their mothers. If large numbers of those babies met regularly, for example at play groups or at day care centres, the chance of transmitting the virus would be increased, as would the likelihood that many of the women were from middle class backgrounds and so less likely to have received protection from CMV acquired in childhood. Overall, Sergio reasoned that changing fashions in breastfeeding and use of day care could markedly affect how many babies were damaged by CMV; he published a paper saying so in the prestigious *Proceedings of the National Academy of Sciences USA.*

In Richmond, Virginia, Stuart Adler had confirmed that CMV was transmitted from toddlers to their mothers and wanted to see if vaccines could interrupt this transmission. Seronegative women were given Towne vaccine or placebo and followed to determine how many would acquire CMV. In parallel, seropositive women were followed in the same way to measure how effective natural immunity was under the same circumstances at preventing reinfection. The results showed that about 10% of seropositive women became infected. The corresponding figure for the seronegative women was almost 50%, irrespective of whether they had received vaccine or placebo. This disappointing result cancelled out the more encouraging results that Stanley Plotkin had seen with Towne vaccine in renal transplant patients. Although the study in Richmond had selected only a low dose of vaccine, it was decided that the substantial financial investment which would be required to develop the vaccine further could not be justified and so work came to a halt.

However, the Richmond study provided an important clue towards the mechanism of action of the vaccine. The amount of cell mediated immunity it induced in seronegative women was similar between those who did or did not become infected, but the amount of antibody was higher in the latter. Furthermore, the seropositive women had much higher levels of antibody than were induced by the vaccine. Stuart's conclusion in the paper was: *"the major finding of this study is the relative protection afforded by a primary infection due to a wild-type virus and the association of this protection with high levels of neutralizing antibodies to* CMV."

Several research groups were conducting experiments with animal versions of CMV. These offered the advantage of being able to directly challenge animals with live virus at a known time and to subsequently collect samples from internal organs to work out what the virus had been doing. However, they had the distinct disadvantages that the viruses were different because mouse CMV had evolved with the mouse and monkey CMV had evolved with the monkey. The viruses also had to be given by injection which did not mimic how human CMV was acquired mainly through kissing.

Although mice and guinea pigs might look similar to the untrained eye, they had an important difference which was relevant to studying CMV. The guinea pig placenta has a similar construction to that of humans so guinea pig CMV can pass through this organ to infect the pups. In contrast, the mouse has a different type of placenta which acts as a barrier to mouse CMV so researchers could not use this model to study congenital CMV. It did have one advantage over the guinea pig model though; the mouse immune system had been studied for so long that there were plenty of reagents available to investigate cell-mediated immunity. The mouse researchers continued to focus on the finer aspects of how mouse CMV interacted with T-lymphocytes and ignored antibodies, CMV in pregnancy and congenital infection.

Meanwhile, researchers Mark Schleiss and David Bernstein in Cincinnati set out to study the guinea pig model and ask if the immune system could control the worst ravages of this infection. They made an antiserum by infecting guinea pigs with guinea pig CMV and then immunising them with purified virus particles. They then gave this antiserum to pregnant dams and challenged them with live guinea pig CMV. As controls, they gave to other animals a different antiserum which lacked any activity against the virus. The results showed that the antibody specific for guinea pig CMV decreased the death rate among pups, although it did not reduce the number of pups which became infected. This result provided a clue that antibody against one or more of the proteins of guinea pig CMV could provide some protection and so opened the door to investigating which component of the virus was important. These results in the guinea pig could be thought of as the animal equivalent of David Snydman's randomised controlled trial of immunoglobulin in transplant patients. Furthermore, they focused attention on the antibody side of the immune system rather than cell mediated immunity which relied on the T cells so familiar to Stevie Headbanger. This was novel, because most other experimenters using animal CMVs were focused on cell mediated immunity.

The gaily coloured hot air balloons sailed over the city every evening, silhouetted against a clear blue sky. The CMV researchers were in Stockholm in May 1995 for the 5th international workshop organised by Per Ljungman. As a clinician performing bone marrow transplants, he no doubt expected to focus on this condition, but his meeting turned out to have the largest attendance to date, about 600, because of the number of cases of CMV retinitis which were affecting AIDS patients.

Researchers in the USA studying the DNA of human CMV noticed some unusual results. When they compared the DNA patterns of CMV strains propagated in the lab with wild-type strains from patients there were obvious differences. The total amount of DNA was the same, but it looked as if the lab strains had lost a segment of DNA and duplicated another piece of DNA to make up the deficit. The researchers conducted a giant molecular jigsaw puzzle to assemble the whole picture and see exactly what pieces were missing from the laboratory-adapted strains. It became clear that approximately 18 genes had been lost from wild-type CMV, about 10% of its total gene content. They advised researchers that the lab-adapted strains were not fully representative of the virus which infected humans. Paul used this information to justify his phrase: *the wrong virus in the wrong cell line using the wrong end point* and thought back to Tom Weller's warning in his review article:

"Several of the established strains of CMV are well adapted to in vitro growth, are widely employed in laboratories around the world, and have been passed many times in tissue culture. Unanswered is the question whether such high-passaged strains of virus have become altered biochemically or antigenically under conditions of prolonged cultivation."

How long should it take for such a perspective from 1971 to filter through into contemporary scientific practice? Why were people still conducting experiments with lab-adapted strains of CMV propagated in fibroblasts a quarter of a century ago?

Chickenpox vaccine was deployed in the USA by giving it to all children with normal immunity. Although Dr Takahashi had developed the vaccine to protect children with leukaemia, the administration of a live vaccine to such children was considered unreasonably risky. Paradoxically then, this new vaccine was recommended for all children except those with immunocompromising conditions like leukaemia.

Although VZV and CMV had been isolated at about the same time by Tom Weller, there was now a licensed vaccine against chickenpox, but still no sign of a CMV vaccine. Of the 5 viruses Tom had isolated, only CMV had not had a vaccine successfully developed. Most researchers considered that it would be impossible to make a vaccine against CMV because of the way it evades immune responses. Others thought that CMV was not important enough to warrant a vaccine, even if one could be made. Instead, CMV disease was slowly being brought under control by preemptive therapy. Most bone marrow transplant centres had simply adopted the technique but one, in Tubingen, conducted a randomised controlled trial to support their decision.

A German haematologist was shocked to see the devastation that CMV could wreak in his patients; even if he had cured their leukaemia, this virus could still kill his patients. He organised a study where patients were randomised to investigation by the standard cell culture technique or by PCR. The results showed that PCR was superior, so providing evidence to support the many groups who had simply adopted this new technique into clinical practice. Slowly, progressively, CMV end-organ disease was being brought under control in transplant patients, although its indirect effects still caused problems.

Matt Williams suddenly felt thirsty. He drank a whole glass of water, but still felt thirsty. His mother gave him a glass of orange squash which helped, but he was thirsty again within the hour. She was worried by this change in his behaviour, took him to see the doctor where diabetes was diagnosed immediately.

Matt integrated into his life the need for insulin to balance his careful diet, but this was difficult when he enjoyed playing sports at school so much. He had a few episodes of fainting, because of low blood sugar and several more where his blood sugar was too high, because he missed an insulin dose to try and give himself more energy for sport. By the time he reached adulthood, it was fair to say that Matt was a poorly controlled diabetic.

The specialists at the hospital warned him that this poor control of blood sugar had damaged his kidneys. They continued to monitor his renal function, but it deteriorated slowly over the next decade, so it was time to discuss further options for him.

"You should consider going on the waiting list for a kidney transplant. You should also consider having a combined kidney and pancreas transplant. This is a rather new technique which doesn't always work but, when it does, can reduce or even eliminate the need for regular insulin injections."

"I'd love to have the chance of cutting down on the insulin routine which has dominated my life since I was a kid. Please put me down for the combined transplant and how long will I have to wait?"

"We never know when a donor will be killed in a car crash. You may never be called or the phone could ring tomorrow."

They did his tissue typing and entered all the details on the national computer. The nurse gave him a pager which he carried with him at all times. If he failed to respond to it, the organ would be offered to the next person on the transplant waiting list who had the right tissue type.

Matt was having a glass of sparkling water to accompany his wife's glass of white wine during a much-needed break from shopping when the vibration in his pocket stopped him in mid sentence. He used his mobile to call the transplant centre and was told to come in immediately without eating or drinking anything. They gathered up their new purchases, retrieved their hatchback from the car park and went straight to the hospital.

There was a lot of hanging about and Matt felt thirsty again, just like he had done as a child when this all started. With drips in his arms and a skimpy white gown on, he smiled at his wife as they wheeled him away.

The double transplant took many hours, but was successful. Matt needed less insulin than before and his new kidney was working perfectly. They let him go home, but that was when stealth virus started to interfere with his new life.

A week later, he developed a fever and went back to the hospital.

"The tests show that you've got stealth virus in your blood. You had this virus when you came to us, so it may be your own virus that's woken up in a process called reactivation. Alternatively, the donor who gave you the kidney and pancreas was also carrying this virus, so it may have come from her. We often see these reinfections with a new strain of virus, but it should respond to treatment."

They gave him some ganciclovir into a vein and watched as the PCR *tests showed the viral load in his blood slowly become negative. He responded to treatment and so did not die from CMV disease, but not before stealth virus had triggered the release of cytokines which damaged his pancreas. Ultimately, Matt's kidney worked well, so he had a much better quality of life, but he never got any benefit from the pancreas transplant and had to return to taking his usual frequent insulin injections because of the indirect effects of a virus he had never heard of.*

Chapter 12: 1997-1999

Results in London explained how preemptive therapy could work so well. By testing serial samples collected twice weekly from patients after transplant by quantitative PCR, Paul and Vince showed that CMV disease occurred only in those who developed a high viral load. This meant that, to be effective at preventing disease, preemptive therapy only had to slow down CMV replication so that it did not reach a high viral load. This was a much more achievable goal than trying to prevent every single case of infection in transplant patients.

Meanwhile, AIDS patients who presented with their first episode of CMV retinitis had moderate to high CMV viral load in the blood which responded promptly to treatment with ganciclovir. When the patients were divided into 2 equal groups, those with the moderate viral load lived longer than did those with a high viral load. The results clearly implied that CMV was hastening the death of AIDS patients, but they couldn't yet measure the viral load of HIV to see if that was the factor responsible for death.

In Alabama, Rich knew that ganciclovir had activity against CMV in AIDS patients from the way in which serial photographs of the retina showed that lesions could be healed if the drug was given. These observations had led to the drug being licensed for CMV retinitis in AIDS patients. Although it was not licensed in children, Rich had decided to conduct a randomised controlled trial to evaluate it in congenital CMV. To minimise toxicity, he had decided to test the possibility that short-term treatment might reduce the viral load and produce clinical benefit even if it could not eradicate CMV completely. If the interpretation of the 1975 paper from Alabama was correct, he might see control of progressive disease even though it was unrealistic to hope for complete control of infection. Treatment for six weeks might be sufficient to test this possibility. Furthermore, he would not assume that the dose chosen for adults was appropriate for babies. He would first do a study comparing two doses and choose the one that gave less toxicity as long as it looked to be equally able to suppress CMV viral load in the urine.

Other doctors had concerns about this proposal. The drug had serious side effects. It would have to be given into a vein, so a surgical procedure to implant a catheter into a deep vein would be needed in newborn infants. These were not simple issues to resolve and the ethics committee deliberated on whether to let the trial proceed. They eventually agreed to do so and, years later, Rich was now looking at the results.

Both doses had produced side effects in about two thirds of cases, requiring the drug to be given at a reduced dose or even stopped in some babies. However, the side effects had been limited to reducing the count of white blood cells, a complication that paediatricians were used to managing. This problem had resolved in all of the children, so that there were no long-term effects on blood. Both doses suppressed CMV in the urine, so there was little to choose between them although the higher dose was perhaps more potent. For the next stage, Rich decided to compare the higher dose against no treatment. Although the study would be randomised, he did not want to subject half the children to a surgical procedure simply to infuse a placebo solution for six weeks. The ethics committee agreed with his decision and Rich recruited a young paediatrician, David Kimberlin, to run the trial.

The pristine white sand ran through the toes of the researchers as they walked along Perdido Beach discussing their favourite virus in March 1997. Bob Pass had organised the 6th international workshop here in the South of Alabama as a perfect way of illustrating the beauty of his State which was much less well-known than the similar attractiveness of its neighbour, Florida. Bob arranged for a keynote lecture to be given by an immunologist from outside the CMV area. As he described how viruses in general could perturb the ability of cell mediated immunity to detect infected cells, it became clear how CMV could establish sanctuary sites within the body where it could replicate free from immunological attack.

Meanwhile, in London, Paul and Vince had completed their quantitative natural history study in renal transplant patients. Patients who were seronegative got primary infection if the donors were seropositive. Such donors could also transmit CMV to patients who were seropositive to cause reinfection. Finally, if the donor was seronegative, then seropositive patients could still reactivate the latent CMV they had brought into hospital.

When Paul and Vince plotted the risk of CMV disease against the peak viral load seen in each patient, a very clear result was obtained. Patients with low or moderate peak viral loads had a minimal risk of CMV disease but, once the viral load passed a certain value, the risk of disease shot up rapidly. They called this transition point the *threshold value* and noted that this was one of the implications of the Alabama paper from 1975. However, there was another factor which correlated significantly with the development of CMV disease; whether the recipient had pre-existing natural immunity to CMV. This was obviously related to the peak viral load, because immunity in the patients could stop CMV replicating to high levels, but which was more important; the presence of immunity or the development of a high viral load?

The classical way of listing factors associated with a condition and determining which were the important ones and which were just the hangers on, was called multivariate analysis. For example, it had been used to study evidence from car crashes which suggested that drivers of red cars were most at risk. In fact, multivariate analysis showed that sports cars were most at risk of crashes and, because they were more likely to be painted red, had led to the false association with car colour. Vince and Paul worked with their statistician colleague Caroline Sabin to perform this clever statistical technique to determine which factor is the prime mover in a relationship and which is simply a fellow traveller. The results were unequivocal; the patients became sick because they had a high viral load. The absence of antibodies in the recipient was statistically significant simply because it was an indirect way of identifying patients destined to have a high viral load after transplant. The results could be explained if CMV established itself in sanctuary sites within the body by expressing its immune evasion genes and continued to pour virus particles into the bloodstream from these sites, so giving the patient a high viral load and a high risk of CMV disease. Vince and Paul incorporated this concept into a model of disease which envisaged CMV passing from one part of the body to another only once a high viral load had been achieved in each of a series of body compartments. Vince and Paul set out to collect more data to put numbers from real patients into their mathematical model.

Once viral load assays for HIV became available, Steve Spector in San Diego performed a multivariate analysis on stored samples from a group of AIDS patients he had recruited previously into a clinical trial. The results showed that the HIV viral load was only marginally associated with mortality, but that an increasing CMV viral load was strongly associated with death. There were no overt signs of a high CMV viral load in these patients and no safe anti-CMV treatment to give them, so clinicians ignored the results.

In Italy, Tiziana Lazzarotto had completed an important study. Italy had started to screen pregnant women for the presence of CMV antibodies as a way of identifying those with recent primary infection. Local laboratories did the initial testing and samples which looked suspicious were then sent on to regional labs like hers. She had evaluated a method for measuring how tightly antibody bound to its antigen which was called the antibody avidity test. Serial blood samples from women with primary CMV infection showed that they took about three months from the time of infection to give high avidity values.

She then showed that women who had CMV before they became pregnant had high avidity antibody and so could be reassured that they had a low risk of having a baby with CMV disease. The risk was not zero, because Sergio's 1977 paper in the *New England Journal of Medicine* had shown that immune women could nevertheless have babies with congenital CMV infection. However, the finding of high avidity was far preferable to being one of the poor women with low avidity, for they had primary infection and so a one in three chance of delivering a baby with congenital CMV. The avidity test was soon established as a reliable technique and was shared widely with other labs in countries which offered to test women for CMV; Belgium and France, but not the USA or UK which would not countenance screening until there was a treatment which could be offered to women who failed the screening test.

Of course, with an infection like CMV which did not produce symptoms, potential treatments could not be evaluated in practice because women were unaware that they were being infected. Introduction of screening tests could be linked to evaluation of potential new treatments, but new treatments would be difficult to study in the absence of screening. The people who made decisions about national screening programmes were different from the people who would evaluate new treatments and neither could act without the other, so the subject stayed in limbo, strung between two bureaucratic empires.

Tiziana also analysed the results of the large number of women who had undergone amniocentesis because of primary CMV infection. Her lab processed the samples looking for

CMV and then she had the difficult task of telling the women which of them was carrying a baby with CMV infection. Tiziana had thought that testing fetal blood by PCR would be more sensitive, but the results showed that amniotic fluid picked up a larger number of positive results.

Another Italian researcher, Maria-Grazia Revello, was working in another regional virology lab providing detailed virology results to confirm or reject the results obtained with screening tests. She was puzzled by a few babies who had been born with CMV in their urine, but where the amniotic fluid had been PCR negative for CMV. She was concerned that the assay had given misleading interpretations to these women and so retested the samples, but continued to get the same results. The amniotic fluid had been taken from women with one of two characteristics; either they had amniocentesis performed before 21 weeks, or they had it done very soon after infection. She reasoned that time must be required for the virus to pass across the placenta and that the fetal kidneys must be fully developed, because amniotic fluid is mainly derived from fetal urine. This result fitted in very well with Tiziana's observation that amniotic fluid was more sensitive than fetal blood for diagnosing congenital infection. More detailed studies would be required to identify and reduce false-positive and false-negative results but, ultimately, the two Italian virologists provided the framework for modern diagnosis of intrauterine CMV infection. Henceforth, women with primary CMV infection who requested diagnostic amniocentesis worldwide would be advised to wait for at least six weeks after the time of presumed infection and until 21 weeks of gestation and would be tested with assays which had become very reliable.

In the same year, Maria-Grazia and her colleagues made an important observation about the way CMV grew in the lab. They were trying to grow CMV in cells that were more representative of the human body than were fibroblasts and experimented with cells from umbilical veins. They could get a few strains to grow, but not all. Eventually, they showed that new isolates of CMV could grow in these vascular cells, but that the lab-adapted strains could not. They wrote their results into a detailed scientific paper in the *Journal of Clinical Investigation* which would become well known.

Bob Pass was committed to controlling congenital CMV infection by vaccination in the way he had seen congenital rubella eliminated from his paediatric practice. It would be difficult to make a live attenuated vaccine against CMV like the type that controlled rubella, because CMV was difficult to grow in the lab. Instead, Bob decided to exploit increasing knowledge about how the immune system responded to viruses. Molecular biology had given us the ability to produce individual protein components of a virus, but these did not elicit strong immune responses when used as vaccines. He knew which protein should be studied first; glycoprotein B, the major protein in CMV that neutralising antibodies bound on to. Glycoprotein B had the major advantage that it was found in all strains of CMV so could potentially provide antibodies that protected against infection with multiple strains. To improve the immune response, the glycoprotein was given with an adjuvant which stimulated the innate immune system. Stimulating the innate and adaptive immune systems at the same time might give good control of CMV. Bob had organised a clinical trial to assess this possibility and was now looking at the results.

Healthy seronegative volunteers had been given three doses of vaccine and the results in front of him showed that their immune systems had responded well. All patients had made antibodies whose quantity was roughly the same as that seen in natural infection. They had a lower level of antibodies which could neutralise CMV infectivity in the lab but, again, these levels were similar to those found after natural infection. Bob wrote up all the results into two scientific papers and set about planning how to immunise women of child-bearing age with this new vaccine. The science was straightforward, but he was astonished to discover the vast amount of paperwork that had to be completed before such a study could be conducted.

Karen Fowler was reviewing the data from the large natural history studies they had performed of CMV and hearing loss to see how many cases would potentially be detected when the new national screening programme for hearing loss was introduced. Her calculations were disappointing, but not unexpected. Many cases of hearing loss caused by CMV were present at birth and so should be detected by the new system which aimed to screen all babies within the first few weeks of life. However, even more babies born with congenital CMV infection had normal hearing at birth but had it damaged progressively over the next few months to years. These cases would not be detected by screening the hearing of neonates, so denying them the opportunity of a diagnosis and underestimating the contribution that CMV made to sensorineural hearing loss.

Again in Alabama, Suresh Boppana was a paediatrician who was preparing to publish his results which he knew would be provocative. He had inherited the role of continuing the natural history studies started by Sergio. This included the 1977 paper showing that immune women could deliver babies born with congenital CMV and the 1992 paper showing that primary infection in the mother represented more of a threat to the fetus than did infection of seropositive women. This latter paper was important, because it showed that, although maternal immunity was not 100% effective, it did offer some protection; indeed, it provided some of the rationale for Bob Pass' attempts to immunise seronegative women. However, the latest results showed Suresh that as many babies with symptoms were born to immune women as were born to seronegative women. As he checked and rechecked the results, he thought of an analogy to explain what, at first glance, could be considered contradictory results in two publications from Alabama.

It was known that women aged 40 years and above had a high risk of having a baby with Down's syndrome. However, so few babies were born to these older women, that 95% of cases of Down's in a population were born to younger women. Despite them, as individuals, having a much lower risk, the abundance of younger women in the population meant that they contributed most cases. In the same way, women with primary CMV infection had a higher risk of having a damaged baby than did seropositive women, but there were so many of the latter in the community that they, as a group, delivered as many babies with CMV disease. Suresh put his manuscript into the envelope to send to *Pediatrics*, anticipating the barrage of letters that the journal would receive once they published it.

Back in London, the results in transplant patients were supplemented by those in further transplant and AIDS patients. When Vince did the maths, he and Paul were surprised at the outcome; the numbers said that CMV was growing very fast in humans, whereas the textbooks emphasised that it grew slowly in cell cultures. It was those cultures again; giving the wrong impression of this virus; *the wrong virus in the wrong cell line using the wrong end point*. Vince then reviewed the results of serial measurements of CMV viral load he and Paul had obtained in AIDS patients. He had used his mathematical skills to calculate the rate at which CMV was replicating and then used this to predict why resistance was slow to evolve among AIDS patients whose CMV retinitis was being treated. They wanted to recruit more patients, but the recent availability of the cocktail of antiviral drugs active against HIV had given many patients back their immunity against CMV and so CMV retinitis was becoming rare; great news for the patients, but bad news for the researchers who would no longer have many cases to investigate.

However, they could look at how well the immune response of these patients performed once the effect of HIV was cancelled by the drug cocktail. Remarkably, AIDS patients rapidly brought their CMV viraemia under control. This explained why they were no longer at risk of getting retinitis, because viraemia was essential if CMV was to reach the eye. It also provided a clue about the types of immune response that controlled CMV because, as well as T-lymphocytes, the amount of antibody against CMV increased when patients were given antiviral drugs active against HIV.

Will I need to bring one of your brollies?

This was a typical e-mail received by Paul just before the 7th international CMV workshop. Britain was famous for its rain, but there was nothing Paul or the organising committee could do about that. They had booked Brighton as the venue for April 1999 and could only hope that the weather would be acceptable for the relatively small number of people who wanted to attend; only 200, no greater than the number who had attended the first workshop in Philadelphia. The problem was that the AIDS doctors had deserted CMV, because it was clear that better control of HIV by means of antiviral drugs also gave better control of CMV.

When the date arrived, the sun did too and stayed for the whole four-day meeting. Those attending did not need a brolly, although a parasol to protect against sunburn would have been appropriate. An immunologist gave an update on new understanding of how T-lymphocytes and components of the innate immune system interacted to destroy cells infected with viruses and how these responses could be impaired by the immune evasion genes of CMV.

Another immunologist in Rochester New York had been investigating immunosenescence. As they get older, many people become short of naive lymphocytes, the type required to respond to new antigens encountered with an infection they have not seen before or a new vaccine, such as the latest seasonal vaccine against influenza. It is known that older people have fewer naive cells because these have been committed to responding to antigens encountered during their long lives. The immunologist wondered if a virus persisting within the host could be presenting antigens repeatedly and so committing many naive lymphocytes to become activated. To test this possibility, antibodies were measured against a variety of viruses in the patients' blood. Remarkably, most of the people with this immunological problem had antibodies to CMV. Furthermore, once CMV was accounted for, the abundance of these cells no longer increased with age and so he questioned the interpretation that they were caused by immunosenescence. This important observation failed to get the attention it deserved because the concept of immunosenescence was so well established and CMV was so poorly understood that this new information was ignored by most researchers.

Edith Morris was frail. Her children and grandchildren paid occasional duty visits to see her, now accompanied by the new generation of great-grandchildren. All the adults were concerned to see her health deteriorate further at each successive visit. She had chronic heart disease and seemed to get a respiratory infection every winter that dragged on for weeks. Her family doctor gave her influenza vaccine every year, but it did not seem to do her any good. The family discussed their concerns with the doctor, but he informed the relatives that there was nothing more he could do.

Unlike James Gordon, Edith had plenty of siblings. They had all acquired the stealth virus when they were young and it had spread in their blood to reach all tissues. Edith was now 87, so she had lived with stealth virus for more than eight decades. She did not know this and neither did her doctor. If he had checked her blood, he would have seen that she was seropositive, but would not have attached any particular significance to this; after all, 60% of people in his practice were in the same category. However, some of these seropositives developed a problem with their immune systems when stealth virus reactivated time and time again and Edith was one of these unfortunate people.

The stealth virus persisted by hiding in sanctuaries within the body that were protected against immune attack by a series of genes encoded within the virus. Each time stealth virus reactivated, the immune system was alerted, but always seemed to be one step behind the virus. Edith's immune system became more and more angry that it could not eradicate stealth virus from those sanctuaries in the way that it had thrown other viruses like measles virus out of her body within two weeks of infection. With time, the immune system committed more and more resources to attacking stealth virus so that, by the age of 87, most of Edith's CD8 lymphocytes were actively searching for the sanctuaries where stealth virus was hiding. Indeed, her body was committing more immune resources to chasing after stealth virus than to all the other viruses combined that she had encountered in her long life.

The effects of this could be put into two distinct categories. First, the CD8 lymphocytes were inflamed and angry that they could not kill stealth virus, so they attacked other tissues instead, including the cells which lined her arteries. This was not the cause of her heart disease, but it contributed significantly to its chronic nature. Second, because most of her lymphocytes were chasing stealth virus, Edith was short of the naïve lymphocytes which were required for her to respond to new antigens, whether found in viruses and bacteria or in the vaccines designed to protect against them. Thus, when her doctor gave her the seasonal influenza vaccine each year, her immune system could not respond. He labelled her as frail with immunosenescence, meaning that her immune failure was simply due to old age. He pursued this conventional medical practice without realising that stealth virus was contributing to the process of ageing of her immune system and hastening her demise.

Although the doctor gave her the annual influenza vaccine as usual that autumn, she failed to respond, developed influenza infection in January and died soon after. He wrote on the death certificate: ***death due to influenza with underlying cardiovascular disease****. He could not add the contribution from stealth virus, because he did not know about it. Neither did any of the family doctors in the UK who filled in the same death certificates for the 500 to 3,000 people who died each* *year from "influenza," most of whom were also infected with stealth virus. Medical researchers responded to this problem by trying to develop newer influenza vaccines which the elderly could respond to, rather than by trying to mitigate the effect of stealth virus on the immune system.*

Chapter 13:
2000-2001

The results had been a long time coming; about a decade to be precise. Paul had a set of data from about 10,000 pregnant women tested for CMV antibodies in a study which started when he was a student. He then had another dataset from about 2,500 pregnant women tested after he went to the Royal Free. The results from the two populations were very similar and the overall interpretation was clear; approximately 58% of women were seropositive at an average age of 26 years. Approximately 2% of seronegatives acquired CMV each year, so the slope of the plot of percentage seropositive against time increased at about 1% per annum. Paul had written up the results into papers for the obstetrics and gynaecology community, but wanted to use the information to address another question. There were very few people who could do the mathematical analyses, but he had met a key researcher at a meeting and proposed a collaboration. She had agreed, but needed to move academic jobs before she would be able to do the analyses. Now that he could see the figures, Paul was not surprised, but had needed the precise mathematical values to make the argument that he knew would be provocative.

Viruses that are highly contagious, like measles, infect people easily, so they catch them early in life. By knowing the average age of infection and the rate of acquisition of infection in a community, one could work backwards and calculate how contagious any given virus must be. This had been done for several viruses, but not for CMV previously. When these viruses were listed according to the average age of infection, it was not surprising that those at the top of the list, like measles, were difficult to control because they were so contagious. It was also not surprising that those at the bottom of the list, smallpox and polio, had either been eradicated from the world by vaccination, or had been scheduled to be eradicated by the World Health Organisation. In fact, there was a clear mathematical relationship, called the basic reproductive number, which linked together the proportion of a community who would need to be protected by vaccination if a virus was to be eradicated. It was this number that Paul had been waiting for and now he could confirm his instinct.

The results were striking: CMV would not be difficult to eradicate once we had an effective vaccine. In fact, if only 60% of a population could be protected from getting primary infection, then CMV would be eliminated within decades from developed countries and potentially eradicated from the globe after that. Numerically, it would be easier to achieve this for CMV than for either smallpox or polio, the two viruses which WHO had so far targeted for eradication. Of course, we did not yet have a vaccine against CMV, but Paul thought he would pave the way for deploying one once it became available just as Sergio's 1975 paper had shown which babies could be treated once a drug was developed years later. Paul wrote the results into a scientific paper with the title: *encouraging prospects for immunisation against primary cytomegalovirus infection* and submitted it to the journal *Vaccine*. The peer reviewers were surprised to see the results, because most people assumed that it would be impossible to make a vaccine against CMV, but the analysis was technically sound, so they recommended publication.

Paul then received a letter inviting him to present these findings at a meeting in Atlanta which was being organised to celebrate the release of a report from the Institute of Medicine. The panel had been charged with identifying unmet medical needs of vaccinology and calculating which infections could justify the expense of developing a vaccine. To the surprise of many, CMV shot up the list to become the vaccine which had the potential to be most cost-effective. Those who worked on CMV were not surprised by this, because they knew how many children (like Rachel Rogers) were damaged by CMV but, for many doctors and scientists, the costs of looking after and educating children with hearing and/or developmental problems were *out of sight, out of mind.* The Institute of Medicine report, using standardised criteria to compare all infections, assessed CMV as a major pathogen for which a vaccine should be developed as a priority.

Paul gave his talk in Atlanta, explained that the virus was spread by contact with saliva, that children were the major source, but that sexual contact could also transmit the virus. He summarised the results showing that a vaccine able to protect 60% of the population would be sufficient to allow eradication through herd immunity. This meant that CMV was not easily transmitted and made sense; after all, the Pope must have met and shaken hands with thousands of people, yet never acquired CMV until he had that single unit of blood as part of a life saving transfusion.

The analysis by the Institute of Medicine was very welcome and would be influential. If reviewers could now be persuaded that CMV was a worthy target for a vaccine, then

Paul knew exactly how to study it in humans. He stayed awake on the flight home drafting out the concept and resolved to contact the manufacturers of the glycoprotein B vaccine that Bob Pass had reported on recently to see if they would provide vaccine for a placebo-controlled trial in transplant patients at the Royal Free. If the answer was yes, he would apply for a grant to obtain the necessary funds. He doubted if this would be possible in the UK, because of the general scepticism about the importance of CMV, and so decided to seek a grant from the USA National Institutes of Health; they should be aware of the report from the Institute of Medicine and be willing to support an initiative, even if it was provocative.

Meanwhile, Mark Schleiss and David Bernstein in Cincinnati had made progress with the guinea pig model of CMV which was difficult to work with, but had the advantage of transmitting virus across the placenta. They reasoned that their earlier encouraging results with an antiserum might be explained if the animals had made antibodies against the glycoproteins which decorate the surface of the virus particles. They therefore purified viruses, extracted the surface glycoproteins and used this preparation as a vaccine to immunise guinea pigs before they became pregnant and kept others as controls. After challenging with live guinea pig CMV, the vaccine decreased the death rate among pups, just as had been seen with the previous antiserum experiment, but also decreased the number of pups born with congenital CMV. Mark and David concluded that the active component in their original antiserum was an antibody made against one or more of the surface glycoproteins of the virus.

In Italy, Maria-Grazia and her colleagues had also taken a step forward in investigating different strains of CMV. They knew that only recent isolates could be cultured in their human vascular cell cultures. They now showed that such isolates lost the ability to grow in the cells if they were cultured repeatedly in fibroblasts. The most likely explanation was that the strains were losing a set of genes required for entry into vascular cells when they were cultured in fibroblasts. Because researchers in the USA had performed a molecular jigsaw puzzle to identify which genes were missing from laboratory adapted strains, it seemed likely that one or more of these genes was normally responsible for allowing CMV to enter into vascular cells. The Italian lab, and several others, set out to identify these key genes and study the proteins they encoded.

The CMV researchers were back in the sand, because Ed Mocarski had organised the 8th international workshop at Asilomar Conference Center on the Monterey Peninsula of California in May 2001. The area of unspoiled natural beauty provided a get away from it all venue conducive for interactive, reflective discussions in buildings constructed in 1913 using the *Arts and Crafts* style. Another meeting had famously been held here in 1975 when pioneers of genetic manipulation met and agreed to a voluntary moratorium on their experiments while rules governing the safety of this new set of techniques were worked out.

Most virologists who changed from working with one virus to another did so to research retroviruses like HIV, because of its medical importance and because funding was more readily available for AIDS. Bill Britt went in the opposite direction; after conducting research on retroviruses, he moved to Alabama to work on CMV, having seen the diseases it caused during his training in paediatrics.

Suresh and Bill had conducted an innovative experiment. It was clear from the work in transplant patients that there were three types of CMV infection; primary, reinfection and reactivation. In the first, patients had no pre-existing immunity. In the second, they had natural immunity, but this could not protect them from an external source of CMV. In the third, they had natural immunity, but this could not protect them from a source of CMV reactivating from within their own bodies. Researchers in London had managed to identify these three types in some selected cases of transplant patients because they had virus to work with and so could type the strains directly. Suresh and Bill suspected that the same three types of infection occurred in women of childbearing age but, in the absence of symptoms to alert them when to look for virus, could only study them in retrospect by looking for the production of antibodies. Their natural history studies informed them that by the time the women made antibodies they would no longer have CMV detectable even when using a sensitive assay like PCR. What they needed was a way of examining the antibody response to determine who had been reinfected among the seropositive women and separate them from the women having reactivations. Those with primary infection would be easy to identify, because they would lack CMV antibodies to begin with and would have low avidity antibody.

CMV has a series of proteins on its surface. Glycoprotein B was one of these and was being evaluated by Bob Pass as a potential vaccine component. Bill had studied the antibody response to other CMV glycoproteins and had noticed that only some women had antibodies against all the parts of glycoprotein H. He reasoned that it must take several infections with different CMV strains before women acquired all of these responses. He and Suresh then designed a study where they would start with babies born with congenital CMV and look back at the serum samples collected from their seropositive mothers. If the women had made new responses to glycoprotein H during pregnancy, Bill and Suresh would classify them as reinfections whereas, if no such responses were seen, they would call them reactivations.

The results showed that the babies born to women who had been reinfected with a new strain of CMV were more likely to have CMV disease than were those born to women who had reactivated their own strain of CMV. This meant that, with time, the immune system had learned to deal with the worst effects of the CMV strain a woman had been infected with in the past, but that this immunity might not protect against another strain circulating in the community. The implication was that a vaccine able to protect against multiple strains might be able to confer substantial benefit. The results also fitted in with those from transplant patients where the severity of CMV could be ranked: primary was worse than reinfection which was worse than reactivation. The scientific paper describing these results, although controversial, was a significant step forward and so the peer reviewers recommended publication in the *New England Journal of Medicine.*

Mary Simpson was an excellent teacher. The pupils in her primary school admired and even worshipped her, while their parents were delighted that the school had recruited such a dynamic young teacher. The headmistress was relieved to have attracted such a committed professional to their school despite its below average rankings in the league tables. Thank goodness that Mary's husband Martin had come to the town to take a good job as a design engineer at the local factory. By all accounts, he should progress up the managerial ladder and would be staying put for several years. Of course, the fact that Mary was married might lead to the headmistress having to advertise to cover maternity leave in the future. Never mind; she shouldn't cross bridges too early and, anyway, it would be better to have Mary temporarily absent than to have to struggle along with a permanent teacher of the usual calibre.

After two years in the town, Martin rushed home to tell Mary that he had been given a promotion. Mary was delighted, but not surprised, because her husband was clearly an accomplished engineer as well as being tall and handsome. They went out to dinner at a country hotel a few miles away to celebrate where conversation inevitably focused on the next stages in their life together. Gazing at each other as the candlelight danced on the empty desert plates, they decided that they would set down roots in the town and start a family.

The headmistress was delighted to see in the latest league table rankings that her school had moved out of the bottom group. She had no doubt that much of this achievement was down to the extremely impressive work of Mary Simpson who was a role model for the other teachers as well as a focus for the parents who were now supporting the school like never before. The knock on her door, which presaged Mary's announcement that she would be going on maternity leave, came as a heavy blow. Full marks to Mary though; she would be absent for only one term, having made child care arrangements able to meet the high standards she expected from all around her.

"I couldn't possibly put my baby in a day care centre. I've seen how children get one runny nose after the other in those places. Although it's much more expensive, I've found a local childminder who will look after my little boy while she cares for her own son. He's just 6 months older than Richard will be so they can play together."

Mary and Martin delighted to see Richard progressing on a daily basis and were so blissfully happy with their new family that they decided to enlarge it as soon as possible. The headmistress had no sooner been relieved to see the end of the supply teacher who covered Mary's absence, than Mary announced that she would, once again, be going on maternity leave.

Richard gave his mummy a big kiss when she came to collect him from the childminder's house and thereby transmitted stealth virus to her. Mary was one of the 60% of the population who had acquired stealth virus as a child and so had good immunity against her own strain. However, just as the immune system could not completely prevent the stealth virus from replicating within a person, it also could not prevent new strains coming from outside to cause a second infection. Such reinfections were common, but did not usually produce any symptoms, because the antibodies and T-lymphocytes did their job and limited the viral load of the stealth virus. Yet, the absence of disease in Mary was not important here; it was the possibility of transmitting stealth virus across the placenta that mattered. Mary was unlucky, for only 1% of women who had natural immunity before they became pregnant delivered babies congenitally infected with stealth virus. Mary's immunity allowed her to remain oblivious to the fact that her placenta and then her unborn daughter were allowing the stealth virus to replicate within. The good news was that Mary's immunity stopped the baby having the most severe types of outcomes such as Sue Rogers and Judith Jones had endured. The bad news was that it couldn't stop her family suffering some ill effects because she now had a different strain which Richard had acquired from the childminder's son.

Mary and Martin called their new daughter Helen and were delighted to see her develop just like Richard had. The little boy doted on his baby sister and Mary looked forward to their happy life together now that her family was complete. She made arrangements to return to work next term and for Helen to go to the same childminder who had looked after Richard so well.

Helen had passed the routine hearing test soon after she had been born but, when she was about eight months old, Mary noticed that Helen did not turn towards sound in the way that Richard had done at that age. Mary went to the GP and arranged to have some hearing tests done. The audiologist told Mary that Helen was moderately deaf in one ear and slightly deaf in the other. It was a type of nerve deafness called sensorineural hearing loss for which there was no treatment. Over the next few months this progressed so that Helen became profoundly deaf on both sides. All the tests that were done had been normal, except for one, which showed that stealth virus was responsible. The audiologist advised it was important that a cochlear implant operation was performed as soon as possible so that Helen's brain could develop in response to sound. She put Helen on the long waiting list for the procedure and advised Mary to learn sign language.

Mary put as much effort and professional commitment into learning sign language and looking after her daughter as she had put into her teaching career. There was no suitable school for children with hearing difficulties nearby so, eventually, she came to the decision that she should stay at home and educate her daughter herself. Martin agreed that they could manage to live on his improved salary. Mary went to see the headmistress to explain why she was resigning and said, truthfully, how much she would miss the school.

Mary bought a little puppy for her children to play with and learn responsibility for another person. When she collected the tiny poodle she was surprised to be given an information sheet saying that the puppy could not meet any other dogs until one week after her second dose of vaccine. Clearly, the vets were more advanced than the medical profession in advising their clients how to avoid common virus infections. If there were vaccines for dogs, why weren't there more for humans to protect them from the risks of normal social contact? If only the doctor had been able to give the childminder's son and Richard a vaccine against stealth virus, Helen might not be suffering from profound deafness.

Helen grew up to be an accomplished young lady who succeeded, despite her disability, because of the commitment her mother made to give her the best chance in life. Although her case may have been recorded in the official statistics describing the damage caused by stealth virus, no one could account for the missed opportunities of the generations of children who attended Mary's old school as it drifted back down the league tables.

Chapter 14: 2002-2003

Another research group in the UK came across CMV from a different angle. Normally, white blood cells reacted to an infection and then died off once the infection was cleared. In some people, there were so many T-lymphocytes of the same type that they formed clones, reminiscent of the cells which ultimately turn into cancerous lymphomas which he saw in his clinical practice. The researchers wondered if a persistent virus might be responsible, looked for evidence of past infection with herpesviruses and found that the people with T-cell clones were all CMV seropositive and so had all had CMV in the past. This chimed with the 1999 results from the USA reporting that a particular type of CD8 lymphocyte was found in people with CMV infection. The haematologists wondered how the virus did that and what medical significance it had.

Michael Boeckh, working in the large bone marrow transplant centre in Seattle, had introduced preemptive therapy for CMV and seen major diseases such as CMV pneumonia largely eliminated. However, it was possible that CMV infection was still triggering the indirect effects first described by Bob Rubin after heart transplantation and so Michael used the results from their large population to investigate this. Supported by the Fred Hutchinson funding, Seattle hosts the largest bone marrow transplant unit in the world, so he was able to analyse results from nearly 2,000 patients. Compared to patients and their donors who were both seronegative for CMV, all other groups had a higher death rate. Some of this was explained by the bone marrow toxicity of ganciclovir plus cases of CMV disease which had not responded to preemptive therapy, but other patients had succumbed to bacterial and fungal infections without the overt presence of CMV. These patients could not be identified from their individual case histories, but only when their cumulative experience was grouped together to form a large cohort. Michael concluded in his paper in the *Journal of Infectious Diseases* that CMV had indirect effects after bone marrow transplant and that steps should be taken to reduce the associated mortality. The mechanism that allowed CMV to do this was not clear, but it could be related to the way this virus diverted immune resources away from the infections they should be controlling; in this case, bacteria and fungi. The observation illustrated how CMV was causing problems behind the scenes without the doctors knowing that this virus was contributing to the illness of their patients.

Back in London, Vince and Paul used their viral load measurements to examine whether transplant patients with prior natural immunity could help control CMV post-transplant. Not only did the immune system make a contribution, it was substantial. The observation provided further support to

Paul's plans to conduct a randomised placebo-controlled trial of the glycoprotein B vaccine in transplant patients and he was delighted to receive a letter from the USA telling him that the grant reviewers at the National Institutes of Health agreed. He set about preparing the vast amount of paperwork required to let such a study be conducted.

Meanwhile, work on the guinea pig form of CMV had also focused on glycoprotein B. Mark Schleiss and David Bernstein wondered if the protective effect of a vaccine containing multiple glycoproteins could be replicated if they immunised with just one of them and chose to study glycoprotein B. They gave a DNA vaccine which made the guinea pigs make antibodies against this glycoprotein. They then gave live virus to pregnant animals and compared their pregnancy outcomes with controls which had not been given vaccine. The results showed a reduced, but not significant, number of deaths among pups accompanied by a significantly reduced number of pups born with congenital infection. They concluded that antibodies against glycoprotein B were a major component of the protective effect of their original antiserum and noted that parallel experiments with a vaccine designed to stimulate cell mediated immunity had not shown any benefits in their guinea pigs. Despite this, most work with other animal CMVs remained focused on the mouse model and was mapping in exquisite detail the cell mediated immune response to mouse CMV, while ignoring humoral immunity.

Karen Fowler also had encouraging results about immunity to CMV. She and Bob Pass had been analysing pregnant women who delivered babies with congenital CMV despite having been seropositive before becoming pregnant. Many people commented that such cases proved it would be impossible to make a vaccine against CMV; if natural immunity was not protective, then how could one hope to produce a vaccine which did better than nature? Karen was concerned that such criticisms were being put in absolute terms: if one such infection occurred then vaccination would be deemed impossible. To provide a comparative group, she selected all women who delivered babies born with congenital CMV after donating a serum sample during a previous pregnancy. She could then work out the risk of congenital CMV for mothers living in the same community who were seronegative or seropositive before they conceived. The results showed that the risk for seronegative women of seroconverting and transmitting virus was high. In contrast, the risk of delivering a baby with congenital CMV was about 69% lower in women who were seropositive. Thus, pre-existing maternal immunity did provide substantial protection to the fetus, although it was not 100%.

Maastricht was the setting for the 9th international CMV workshop organised by Cathrien Bruggeman and colleagues in May 2003. This collegiate town of cobbled streets provided an excellent venue to discuss the research that had gone on since the researchers had last met in Asilomar. It was also an appropriate location for the researchers to grumble to each other about the impending wave of bureaucracy which was being proposed by the European Union to regulate the conduct of clinical trials. A keynote lecture focused discussions on the inflammatory nature of atherosclerosis and how some of the genes of CMV could be responsible for accelerating this disease process.

In Alabama, David Kimberlin and Rich were looking at the long-awaited results of their study. A proportion of the children born with symptoms who were randomised to no treatment had developed hearing loss and developmental delay typical of congenital CMV. In contrast, the children given ganciclovir had developed side effects, but these were manageable, even though about a third of the babies had required the dose to be reduced. Importantly, the drug protected the babies' ears against further damage from CMV. Although it did not repair much of the damage that CMV had already done to structures within the inner ear and did not abolish all hearing loss, the effect was so important that a six-week treatment course was recommended for any baby who was born with the symptoms and signs listed in the protocol. Thus, this treatment became accepted worldwide as the standard of care for symptomatic congenital CMV infection even before the paper was formally published, because CMV specialists had been eagerly awaiting the results and were impressed when David presented them at scientific meetings.

Penny Abbott listened to the words that the doctor was saying. She could tell that he was trying to be kind and break bad news to her gently, but couldn't take in the details. She knew that her newborn son Nathan didn't look as healthy as her daughter Judy had done when she was only 2 days old. The tubes taped to Nathan, which dived into his tiny little body at several different places, didn't help. She thought of so many questions, anticipated so many problems, but could only form the briefest of sentences to convey her overwhelming sense of foreboding:

"Will Nathan get better?"

The doctor knew that the prognosis in these cases of congenital stealth virus infection was notoriously difficult to predict. Some did really badly and were left with major neurological problems, while others seemed to fight off the worst ravages of infection.

"It really is too soon to say, Mrs Abbott. The tests show that Nathan's head is much smaller than it should be, so we're concerned about how he'll develop. The test tomorrow will tell us if his hearing has been damaged. The other symptoms; the yellowness of jaundice and the skin rash, should get better over the next few weeks."

"Is there any treatment?"

For the last case he saw, about a year ago, he had to give a negative response, but now he could be a bit more optimistic.

"Some paediatricians in the USA have just reported an important study with babies like Nathan. They gave half of them a drug called ganciclovir for 6 weeks and observed the other half. When they repeated the tests 6 months later, the babies given the drug were less likely to have hearing loss. The drug has side-effects and has to be given into a vein, but we recommend that you consider letting Nathan have a course. He looks just like the other babies in the USA trial and so should get some benefit. However, it's not realistic to expect the drug to repair any damage that's already occurred; its main effect is to protect the hearing against further damage."

"We want to give Nathan every chance, so please go ahead."

The doctor left to see when the surgeons could implant a catheter into the little boy's body to allow the drug to be infused into a deep vein. He thought how lucky he was to work in the NHS, where his signature on a prescription form would be sufficient to justify giving this new treatment to his patient. Ironically, paediatricians in the USA, where the trial had been conducted, were having difficulty prescribing ganciclovir, because health insurance companies had not yet agreed to pay for the drug.

Nathan responded to treatment by not developing hearing problems. He still had difficulties meeting all his developmental milestones, but the local school said he could stay there with his friends, rather than needing special attention at a distant school for children with both hearing and neurological problems. Penny still had challenges looking after Nathan, but the doctor was pleased to see that the little boy was doing better than the last case he had seen. Slowly, some of the worst effects of stealth virus were starting to come under control.

Chapter 15:
2004-2005

It was a research collaboration from Italy and Germany which identified the three extra genes required for CMV to enter cells of the vascular system. As expected, these three genes were among the 18 which were lost when CMV was cultured in fibroblasts, harking back to Tom Weller's warning in 1971 that the strains of CMV adapted to cell culture might not be representative of the real CMV. Each gene produced a single protein and all three proteins had to be present together to allow CMV to bind on to vascular cells and to enter them.

In fact, other proteins were involved as well because researchers in the USA showed that these three novel proteins interacted with two known glycoproteins (one of which was glycoprotein H) to form a five-member complex responsible for entry into vascular cells. At last, lab work on CMV in cell cultures could move on from studying *the wrong virus in the wrong cell type* and could determine how this virus affected cells of the vascular system and so potentially understand how it increased the risk of atherosclerosis. As well as improving understanding of CMV biology, any of these five proteins could now be considered as potential components of a new vaccine against CMV.

Meanwhile, the researchers in Cincinnati had more evidence that glycoprotein B was important as a component of a CMV vaccine. They immunised guinea pigs with glycoprotein B together with an adjuvant to stimulate the innate immune system. All animals made good antibody responses to the vaccine, especially those given the adjuvant. Once the animals were pregnant, they were challenged with live virus and monitored for the outcome of pregnancy. This time, significant reductions were seen in both the death rates of pups and in the proportion born with congenital infection. Mark Schleiss and David Bernstein concluded that antibodies were important, that glycoprotein B was important and that an adjuvant was important. They said so in a paper published in the *Journal of Infectious Diseases*, but investigators with mouse and monkey models of CMV continued their focus on cell mediated immunity and ignored the antibody response.

Paul was invited to give a talk at a meeting of transplant physicians. The next speaker gave an interesting description about the register she kept of infections reported from throughout the USA which were acquired during the process of transplantation. She gave a long list of infections, each with cases numbered in single digits per year, but did not mention CMV until it came time for questions:

"What about all the cases of CMV?"

"Oh, we couldn't possibly keep track of all of those. By convention, we don't list the cases of CMV because it's just routine for that virus to be acquired from the donor."

No wonder people failed to acknowledge the importance of CMV in transplantation if the body charged with recording the number of cases had to ignore this virus because there were just too many to keep up with.

Karen Fowler and Bob Pass performed another analysis on their cohort of pregnant women to address a medically important question. When a woman had a baby with congenital CMV infection, she had to try to understand its complex natural history. Frequently, she would then ask when it would be safe to have another pregnancy. Karen's analysis showed that the immune system took time to get to grips with CMV but, eventually, the rate of congenital CMV in subsequent pregnancies declined towards its baseline value. There was never a time when a seropositive woman could have a pregnancy guaranteed to be free from congenital CMV but, about one year after the presumed time of infection, the risk was no longer excessive, so she could plan for another pregnancy. This timing corresponded to at least two years between the births of the siblings.

CMV experts throughout the world read Karen's paper and adapted the advice to women according to their personal circumstances. It was particularly difficult for those few women who had been advised to have a termination of pregnancy because CMV had caused extensive fetal damage revealed by ultrasound scans. Typically, they came from middle-class backgrounds, had avoided CMV as a child and so entered their childbearing years without immunity against CMV. Often, they were professionals who had delayed their first pregnancy until their careers were established and had acquired primary infection during their second pregnancy while their firstborn attended day care. They now had to wait longer than anticipated to complete the family they had planned and felt their biological clocks ticking as the months passed.

The CMV experts wished they had an intervention which could speed up this process, but had nothing to offer. It was possible that a vaccine could be given to such women to accelerate the development of immunity to CMV, but this would require a clinical trial. It would also need to use the vaccine for immunotherapy; that is, providing benefit by administering vaccine to people who have already been infected in the past. No controlled clinical study had ever been conducted to determine if vaccines could be used in this way. Paul's study of giving vaccine or matching placebo to patients awaiting transplant would address this possibility by studying seropositive as well as seronegative people, but was still tied down in bureaucracy two years after the paperwork had first been submitted. The new law foreshadowed at the Maastricht meeting had been introduced from Europe which created a massive, detailed process for conducting randomised controlled trials. The stated aim was to improve patient safety, but it was very unlikely that this would be achieved. Instead, it would have the effect of delaying access to potential new treatments. The newly created army of bureaucrats required to administer this scheme had no sense of urgency so, at this rate, Paul's study would take longer to obtain approval than it would to conduct the three-year clinical trial.

Paul did however have some results to look at; those from the first randomised controlled trial to evaluate combination antiviral treatment for CMV. They knew that two drugs, ganciclovir and foscarnet, when studied in fibroblast cell cultures in combination, inhibited CMV better than would be expected if the effect of one drug was simply added to the effect of the second. If such synergy could be demonstrated in humans, it would be important because it would give more rapid control of CMV. Furthermore, it should reduce the side effects of treatment, because ganciclovir is toxic to the bone marrow whereas foscarnet is toxic to the kidneys. By sharing out the toxicity and giving each drug at half the normal dose, such combination therapy could be more tolerable for patients than was ganciclovir alone.

To study the possibility of synergy in humans, the team in London recruited transplant patients who needed preemptive therapy. Instead of giving them all a standard course of ganciclovir, they randomised them to receive the standard ganciclovir or ganciclovir at half dose plus half dose foscarnet. The study had gone well, but the results were disappointing. Not only was there no evidence of a synergistic effect, there was a strong trend in favour of ganciclovir alone being more potent and better tolerated than the combination. While the results failed to demonstrate synergy, they illustrated, again, that the culture of lab adapted strains of CMV in fibroblasts often gave misleading results; *the wrong virus in the wrong cell line using the wrong end point.*

However, the London lab did have some positive results; in AIDS patients this time. When combination antiviral therapy against HIV was introduced, it rapidly brought HIV under control and partially repaired the damage that this virus had done to the immune system. The normal count in the blood of the CD4 helper T-lymphocytes that Stevie Headbanger had been told about was 1,000 and opportunistic infections such as CMV typically occurred once the count dropped below 100. If a new set of antiviral drugs active against HIV could be started at this time, then the risk of CMV disease decreased soon after the CD4 count went back above 100. The introduction of potent combination treatment for HIV had been so spectacularly successful that CMV retinitis was now an uncommon condition. Several AIDS physicians joked that Paul should find another virus to work on because CMV had disappeared from their patients. This annoyed him, because they appeared not to be aware that CMV was also a major pathogen for the fetus and for transplant patients. It also annoyed him, because it was an assumption without any evidence to back it up; the disease CMV retinitis had gone away, but CMV infection could still be common in their patients. If so, it might still be exerting its indirect effects. Deciding to diplomatically avoid the word *cofactor* which had so antagonised the AIDS physicians a decade earlier, Paul decided to conduct a natural history study looking for CMV infection because, guided by the advice in Tom Weller's review, CMV was such a wily opponent that nothing about it should be accepted until it had been proven.

The protocol was simple in design but sophisticated in its analysis of every patient with HIV at the Royal Free whose CD4 count had ever been below 100. Every time these patients came to the clinic to have their CD4 count and HIV viral load measured, another sample was taken to measure CMV by PCR. After three years of follow-up, Caroline Sabin performed state-of-the-art multivariate statistical analyses. The researchers were interested in CMV retinitis as an example of CMV disease. They were also interested in measures of the indirect effects of CMV in this patient population which could be assessed in two ways. When AIDS was first described, there were no tests available for HIV because it had not been discovered yet. The disease AIDS was diagnosed when patients like

Billy Rogers had at least one opportunistic infection or tumour from a long list which indicated that they had profound suppression of their T-lymphocytes. This list comprised the *AIDS defining conditions* and would act as one good way of assessing whether CMV was acting as a cofactor to increase the rate at which HIV was damaging the immune system. The second measure was death, because nobody could really argue against the importance of CMV if it killed patients.

When the results were finally available, in summary, detection of CMV by PCR was strongly associated, as expected, with the development of CMV retinitis. However, it was also associated with the occurrence of new AIDS-defining conditions and with death. Indeed, for the latter end point, once the CD4 count and presence of CMV had been accounted for statistically, the HIV viral load had nothing more to add. When Paul presented these results to AIDS physicians he asked why they continued to measure HIV viral load in such patients instead of measuring CMV which identified patients at imminent risk of death. He never received a satisfactory answer to this question, but noted that the AIDS physicians continued with their clinical practice and ignored CMV. It was clear that clinicians focused on what they could see, rather than what they could measure; no wonder CMV was managing to keep out of the limelight.

Paul wanted to design a randomised controlled trial to determine if treatment for CMV could reduce deaths, but Caroline advised that thousands of patients would be needed because very few AIDS patients died each year now that potent anti-HIV therapy was available. Thus, just as in the early phase of the AIDS epidemic, patients with AIDS who died despite receiving the best available therapy did so <u>with</u> CMV, but we would never know if they died <u>because</u> of CMV.

The results were considered worthy of publication in the *Lancet* and the paper ended with the suggestion that a randomised controlled trial of a drug active against CMV should be conducted to see if it could reduce mortality. When Paul showed the results at meetings, he commented that this conclusion was identical to that concluding their 1989 paper in the *Lancet* and stated that he found this lack of attention for 15 years to an important medical problem to be unacceptable. Despite publication of the results in the *Lancet* and repeated pleas for this observation to be followed up, no follow-up study could be performed until an intervention safer than ganciclovir became available.

Ten years after the VZV vaccine was recommended for all children as part of routine immunisation, the CDC (Centers for Disease Control and Prevention) published a paper in the *New England Journal of Medicine* showing that deaths due to chickenpox had been reduced by 66%. The chickenpox vaccine had saved the lives of young children and of adults who would otherwise have come in contact with them. This illustrated clearly that children were the source of this herpesvirus but that disease affected everyone in the community. The parallel with childhood CMV infection causing heartbreak for their pregnant mothers was striking, but there was still no sign of a licensed CMV vaccine.

Latent VZV reactivated to cause zoster or shingles when patients' cell mediated immunity declined. It was suspected that exposure to chickenpox periodically boosted cell mediated immunity so that the development of shingles was delayed. The evidence for this came from paediatricians who were reputed not to develop shingles because of their repeated exposure to chickenpox. Likewise, adults with children in their families had a significantly lower risk of shingles than those without children. Thus, shingles could be predominantly a disease of the elderly because of immunosenescence and/or because elderly people were less likely to encounter chickenpox.

Mike Oxman in San Diego designed a study to test this directly. He recruited more than 38,000 people over 60 years of age and randomised them to receive the Oka strain of VZV vaccine or a matching placebo. Once this massive study was complete, the vaccine had halved the incidence of zoster and the nerve pain associated with it. The study was a great clinical success and was the first scientific demonstration of the concept of immunotherapy. This landmark paper was published in the *New England Journal of Medicine.*

As Paul read the article, he wished that his vaccine study would start, because half of the people on the waiting list for transplant were CMV seropositive and he was planning to boost their immunity against CMV. There was no sign of a start date, because of the new European rules for clinical trials which had effectively stopped investigator-led studies such as his. He had now written three consecutive annual reports to the National Institutes of Health explaining that, although he had responded immediately to every new piece of paperwork, he still did not have permission to start the study. He thought how unethical the imposition of these new rules had been in practice, but was powerless to influence the new bureaucracy. Fortunately, the National Institutes of Health were very understanding and kept the grant open.

A team of immunologists in the USA published a paper which was truly heroic in the amount of effort put into it. They had set out to determine which proteins of CMV the immune system responded to. The answer was that it responded to all of them. Clearly, CMV did not evade immune responses by impairing their induction; instead, it allowed these responses to be produced but then hid from them. This fitted in very nicely with the model of pathogenesis proposed by Paul and Vince which imagined CMV persisting and replicating in sanctuary sites. It also supported the prospect of developing effective vaccines against CMV, because the virus would not be committing so much of its genome to producing immune evasion genes if those immune responses did not represent a threat to it.

The researchers watched the people clad in 18th-century clothing as they went about their daily activities. Colonial Williamsburg was the setting for the 10th international CMV workshop in April 2005 and Stuart Adler had encouraged those attending to see at first hand how tough life had been in the colonies. He asked Paul to chair one scientific session, so allowing the latter to declare that this part of Williamsburg would, once again, revert to British rule if only for the next 2 hours.

Back in Alabama, analysis of the paediatric cohort identified a marker of poor prognosis in neonates with congenital CMV infection. The detection of CMV in the urine or saliva diagnosed congenital infection, but not all babies also had CMV in the blood. Those that did have viraemia had an increased risk of developing hearing loss. This was consistent with the model of several body compartments each controlling CMV which Paul and Vince had proposed. Presumably, babies able to keep CMV infection limited to the urine had better immune control than did those with viraemia. If so, this good immunity may be working to control CMV replication in the inner ear. This observation supported the concept that CMV replication after birth, presumably in the inner ear, was responsible for progressive hearing loss; it also supported the attempts by David Kimberlin and Rich to control this damage by giving antiviral treatment soon after birth. Although they were being cautious by restricting the toxic drug ganciclovir to babies born with symptoms to begin with, one could imagine in the future recruiting children with CMV viraemia but no symptoms to determine if a benefit on hearing could be obtained in this group to offset its undoubted production of side effects. Of course, this would require babies to be screened for congenital CMV and there was no sign of this anywhere in the world.

Although disease caused by CMV clearly had a public health perspective, the CDC in the USA had not become involved in studying it, perhaps because there were other infections of major importance, like HIV and influenza, which took precedence. That perspective changed in 2005 when Mike Cannon and Sheila Dollard, an epidemiologist and a virologist familiar with studying infections at the population level, decided to get involved. They reviewed the published information about congenital CMV and were surprised that this virus seemed to be flying below the public health radar so decided to set up a series of studies to address how CMV might be affecting the public and put it into perspective. Mike Cannon showed that women of childbearing age rarely took routine precautions to protect themselves against acquiring CMV. This would only require them to kiss children in a way that avoided saliva and to wash their hands with soap and water after wiping away saliva or changing babies' nappies and so should not disrupt normal family life excessively. He also found that doctors who took care of such women rarely volunteered information about CMV and how to avoid it. His article: *washing our hands of the CMV epidemic* harked back to the 1972 editorial by Martha Yow in style and berated clinicians for ignoring this important pathogen, emphasising that ***women deserve to be informed*** about the risks that CMV poses during pregnancy.

"Would you ladies mind completing a research questionnaire while waiting for the doctor? We want to know which diseases you think are important in pregnancy."

Mandy Evans looked up to see the pretty, blonde, smiling, slim research nurse standing next to her. Keep away from men and stay that way for as long as possible thought Mandy, as another wave of nausea passed over her and she reflected on how much weight she had put on so far. No need to be grumpy towards the nice nurse came the reply in her head.

"Of course, love; have you got a pen?"

Five minutes later, Mandy regretted her decision. The form was asking about lots of different diseases, but she couldn't quite remember which was which. Come on girl, she thought to herself; remember what was in that booklet they gave you at the first antenatal clinic visit.

She had definitely heard of rubella, so put a tick next to that one. She was fairly sure that Down's syndrome was the one she'd had the tests for, so ticked that one also. There was lots of publicity about not drinking during pregnancy, so she could easily guess that fetal alcohol syndrome was a bad thing. But what was this other condition with the long name? It was written cytomegalovirus (CMV), but she was sure she had never been told about that. It could not be too important if she had never heard about it, so she left that box blank.

Chapter 16:
2006-2008

Maria Barbi, another virologist in Italy, published a paper showing that she could detect CMV DNA in blood reconstituted from dried blood spots which are routinely collected from all neonates to screen for metabolic diseases. This was important for two reasons.

First, it would allow retrospective diagnosis of congenital CMV. If a baby like Helen Simpson presented at 8 months of age with both hearing loss and CMV one could never be sure if the former had been caused by the latter. This was important, because only congenital CMV caused damage to the ears and brain. Although CMV was often acquired from breast milk in the first weeks of life, this did no harm. If we wanted to focus treatment on babies with congenital CMV, we would need a way to exclude cases of infection which were acquired after birth. Now, with this new method, when a baby failed a hearing test their dried blood spot could be retrieved from storage and tested for CMV DNA. If positive, it would represent clear evidence of congenital infection and so indicate that CMV really was the cause of the hearing loss.

Second, the dried blood spots were collected and processed already for the diagnosis of approximately 27 metabolic conditions. Potentially, one could add CMV to this list and so create a national screening programme. Unfortunately, the dried blood spots were not processed by PCR for metabolic screening, so a change of technique would be required. Because much of the cost of a screening programme resides in the infrastructure rather than in the testing itself, the incremental cost of adding CMV PCR onto an existing programme would be lower than proposing a stand-alone system, even if it did require development of a new method.

However, it remained to be determined how sensitive testing for CMV DNA in dried blood spots was. Maria had reported 100% sensitivity, but this seemed unrealistically high, especially given the recent report from Alabama that only some babies had viraemia. Nevertheless, the fact that the presence of viraemia was a marker of poor prognosis, suggested that testing dried blood spots might create a good screening test because the objective was not to find all cases, but to identify those at risk of hearing loss so that they could be offered treatment. Since only 25% of babies born with congenital CMV ultimately developed disease and because those who did so tended to have viraemia and higher viral loads, an insensitive test for detecting infection could nevertheless be useful for finding those at risk of developing disease. Clearly, much more work from large cohort studies would be required to evaluate the full implications of dried blood spot testing.

Vince's original method for quantifying CMV DNA had been useful, but too cumbersome for routine use. Now, new technology had been developed to allow quantitative results to be made available on either the same day or the day after a sample was collected. The lab in London had just moved to testing all samples by this new method of real-time quantitative PCR when Paul finally got permission to start the vaccine study. The availability of real-time results would simplify the data analysis and provide clinically important levels of this CMV biomarker to all patients, not just those in the vaccine trial. Instead of attending the weekly transplant ward rounds to discuss which patients were PCR positive and what the viral loads had been last week, Paul would have up-to-date quantitative results at his fingertips.

The PCR technique had come a long way since Kary Mullis had won the Nobel Prize for describing the concept. A heat resistant polymerase had been discovered in an organism living in hot water and had been cloned to provide the world's labs with a useful reagent so that technicians no longer had to open the tubes after each round of PCR to replace the enzyme that had been damaged by heat. Furthermore, nobody now had to open the tubes to measure the PCR products; instead, clever chemistry was used to produce light every time the polymerase completed a round of replication. This light was stimulated by a laser and captured by a charge-coupled device, similar to that found in digital cameras, through the transparent wall of the reaction tube. This vast improvement in diagnosis owed as much to process engineering as to biochemistry, illustrating how people from different scientific backgrounds could collaborate to solve major problems in medical research.

Mike Cannon decided to see how much the general public knew about CMV and whether they realised that simple precautions like washing hands after changing babies' nappies and avoiding saliva when kissing and hugging them could reduce acquisition of this virus. The results showed that public knowledge about CMV was lower than it was for other infectious agents, because only 22% of women of childbearing age had heard of CMV. Compared to 9 other conditions which could affect the baby, women's awareness was lowest for CMV, despite the fact that this virus caused at least as much disease as the next candidate; fetal alcohol syndrome. In fact, pregnant women were routinely given advice about fetal alcohol syndrome and toxoplasmosis, but not about CMV. Women were offered screening for rubella, spina bifida and Down's syndrome in early pregnancy, but not for CMV, despite it damaging more babies than any of these other conditions.

When encouraging antenatal screening for CMV antibodies, Tiziana had been criticised because people said it would inevitably lead to an increase in the number of women requesting termination of pregnancy. This was a big issue in Italy because of its Catholic heritage, so needed data to inform the debate.

Tiziana showed that most women referred to her for diagnosis decided to continue with the pregnancy if her specialised tests showed that their risk of congenital CMV was no greater than background. Some women whose amniotic fluid was PCR positive did opt for termination of pregnancy, but not those whose result was PCR negative. Overall, the access to specialised tests led to fewer terminations than would have been expected if obstetricians advised women with abnormal screening tests for CMV to have a termination of pregnancy just in case. Thus, the major threat to the fetus was the obstetrician; so Tiziana published her analysis in the *American Journal of Obstetrics and Gynecology* to stimulate discussion.

As the plane came in to land, one of the new iconic aircraft was parked at the side of the runway. By the time the pilot had brought the little Airbus to a walking pace, another of its giant stablemates had come into view. No fare-paying passengers had yet flown on these brand-new beasts, but that would change within months as the A380 double-decker aircraft set out from this, their base, to begin service with airlines all around the world. The 11th international CMV workshop was being held here in Toulouse in May 2007 at a truly historic time for aviation.

It was a historic time also for the CMV field which had taken to heart many of the developments in molecular biology which allowed important scientific questions to be answered. Ed Mocarski gave a lecture explaining how CMV contained a set of proteins which it used to stop a cell dying after it was infected. This allowed the cell to produce new daughter viruses for a long time, in contrast to infections like polio which killed the cell rapidly and so had only a short time to transmit viruses on to other cells and maintain the infectious process. This new insight, together with earlier explanations of how CMV-infected cells evaded the immune system, showed how this virus could persist long term in its host. However, on reaching the airport for their return flights, the researchers had a striking reminder of how innovation was bringing benefits to travellers quicker than to patients suffering from CMV.

The results from the CDC were flowing fast now. Sheila Dollard published a systematic review summarising all the scientific papers from around the world which had looked at the effects of congenital CMV. She could show that about 12% of babies with congenital infection had symptoms at birth and another 13% developed them for the first time when followed up, so that CMV ultimately damaged 25% of those born with congenital infection. Overall, one third of babies who ultimately suffered from CMV had symptoms at birth, while two thirds appeared to be normal and were only identified because they were being actively screened at birth. This explained why congenital CMV was so frequently underestimated by health care systems, because babies were only followed in this way if they were part of a research study.

Mike Cannon published another analysis showing that the rates of congenital infection in different populations around the world could be partly explained by the proportion of people who were infected in each community. This implied that some women must be being reinfected with new strains of CMV, despite having naturally acquired immunity, and subsequently passed CMV onto their unborn babies.

Six years after Paul had published the calculation of the basic reproductive number of CMV, Sheila Dollard and Mike Cannon at the CDC confirmed and extended the results. Using samples from the large, world-renowned National Health and Nutrition Examination Survey (NHANES), they concluded that protection of only 50% of the population by vaccination would be sufficient to allow eradication of CMV, so their results were even more optimistic than Paul's estimate of 60%. They estimated that 27,000 pregnant women in the USA develop primary CMV infection each year. There were now sufficient cases to document the infection risk to the fetus as

1 in 3 instead of 1 in 2 but, although only one third of these infections crossed the placenta, this added up to approximately 9,000 babies born with congenital infection each year.

Back in London, 31 years after he had first visited Alabama, Paul at last got the results he had been waiting for. He had wanted to devise a lab method which did not rely upon cell culture to quantify CMV in newborn babies and relate the values to those who got hearing loss. He had used the quantitative PCR assay for some time now and had shown that the implications of the 1975 paper were true in transplant patients. However, he had never been able to collect a set of samples from children with hearing loss. Paul had a long-term collaboration with Mike Sharland, a paediatrician specialising in infectious diseases at St George's Medical School. Although this was in South London, miles away from the Royal Free in North London, the collaborators were linked by a single underground line which gave the group their informal name: *the Northern Line Researchers.*

A medical audiologist, Simone Walter, came to Mike Sharland looking for a project on CMV, because she knew that his paediatric infectious disease practice specialised in CMV. Mike and Paul put together a study which would eventually get Simone a distinction in her MSc degree. Following on from Maria Barbi's paper, Simone identified known cases of congenital CMV with hearing loss and retrieved their dried blood spots for testing by quantitative PCR using a method developed by Claire Atkinson in Paul's lab. When the code was broken, there was a strong association between the viral load in the dried blood spots and the severity of the hearing loss. Not all children known to have congenital CMV had been detected, but 70% had, meaning that the test would become a useful, although not perfect, way of diagnosing infection that had occurred in the past. However, Paul was more interested in the shape of the curve when the severity of hearing loss was plotted against the viral load in the blood. As he had hoped, it was not a straight line, but followed the *threshold* shape, with a minimal risk at low viral loads and then a sudden transition to high risk. This observation validated the implications of the 1975 paper from Alabama, provided the missing link showing that the model of CMV pathogenesis proposed by Paul and Vince applied to all patient groups affected by this virus and explained why the short six-week course of ganciclovir pioneered by David Kimberlin and Rich had been so successful.

When coupled with detailed knowledge of the ways the immune evasion genes of CMV worked, this new information meant that disease caused by CMV hiding in its sanctuary sites was susceptible to antiviral therapy. Now that researchers knew this, how could they treat more cases for longer than 6 weeks when ganciclovir had to be given into a vein?

David Kimberlin and Rich met to go over the results from their latest study.

They had been encouraged by the finding that six weeks of ganciclovir reduced hearing loss, but wanted to improve outcome even further. The fact that such a short treatment duration provided benefit was based on the 1975 paper from Alabama and the model of pathogenesis proposed by Paul and Vince. The beneficial effects of such a short treatment validated them both. The obvious next step was to give treatment for longer, but this would require an oral drug.

An oral prodrug of ganciclovir, called valganciclovir, had been made by sticking the natural amino acid valine onto ganciclovir. Valine was taken up from the gastrointestinal tract by transporter proteins so, potentially, any drug tagged onto it could be taken up also by piggyback. The prodrug had been developed for adults and required an enzyme in the liver to cleave the prodrug to release valine and ganciclovir into the bloodstream. They could not assume that this enzyme was active in neonates, but could do a study to determine if it was. When children needed six weeks of intravenous ganciclovir as standard of care, they substituted oral valganciclovir at different doses for one or two days and measured the blood levels of ganciclovir. The results showed that the enzyme needed to release ganciclovir from valganciclovir was active in neonates and that they had found a dose which gave the same blood levels as did an intravenous infusion of ganciclovir. They wrote up the results for a specialised pharmacology journal and planned a study to use valganciclovir to see if treatment for longer than six weeks could provide additional benefits. They invited Mike Sharland and Paul to join in the study by recruiting suitable cases from paediatricians in the UK and began the long process to get approval from the clinical trials bureaucracy.

Sheila Dollard and Mike Cannon at the CDC published an analysis of the NHANES dataset relating CMV infection to sexual activity by linking the presence of CMV antibodies with the self-reported assessment of sexual activity and the presence of antibodies against another virus which is known to be sexually transmitted. The results showed a significant association between CMV infection and sexual activity. However, this association explained less than half of all CMV infections, so something other than sexual contact must be the predominant route of transmission of this virus to women of childbearing age. Contact with the saliva and urine of young children was an obvious candidate, so the main conclusion of this paper was that most women of childbearing age acquired CMV infection from children rather than from their consorts. This came as no surprise to paediatricians familiar with CMV, but would require non-specialists to play down their assumption that CMV was frequently transmitted by sexual intercourse.

Meanwhile, Michael Boeckh in Seattle received the results from a randomised controlled trial conducted in bone marrow transplant patients in many cities. A new drug active against CMV called maribavir had the distinct advantage over ganciclovir of lacking toxicity for the newly engrafted bone marrow. Patients had been randomised to receive one of three doses of the new drug or a matching placebo in a proof of concept study. The results showed that maribavir controlled the appearance of viraemia better than did placebo, with no obvious difference between the three doses. The company making the drug was encouraged to develop it further by conducting a large definitive study which could lead to maribavir getting a licence to be prescribed by physicians if the study showed the drug to be both safe and effective.

Another group of investigators led by Michael Boeckh reported interesting findings in a completely different group of patients. There were reports of patients who had been in intensive care for a long time being found to have CMV viraemia. These investigators conducted a systematic study to define the natural history of CMV viraemia in patients who required admission to intensive care units.

A total of 120 seropositive patients were recruited because they needed intensive care following trauma, heart attack, burns or serious medical problems. The researchers collected blood twice a week to look for CMV viraemia and recorded how long the patients stayed in hospital. The results showed that those with viraemia were significantly more likely to need care in intensive care units for extended periods of time.

These results were exciting, but there was a potentially trivial explanation for this important observation; if samples were collected repeatedly, then those who were sampled for longer because they remained in hospital would have a greater chance of having CMV detected if it reactivated intermittently. They examined this possibility by doing a statistical test restricted to those who were still in hospital 30 days after their admission. This so-called landmark analysis excluded the trivial explanation and so provided evidence that CMV might be the cause of the additional stay in the intensive care unit. The results were so compelling that they designed a double-blind, randomised placebo-controlled trial to determine if ganciclovir given to seropositive patients soon after admission to intensive care could reduce the duration of their hospital stay. When the results of the study become available around 2015, they could have a profound impact on medical practice.

Dave Bennett never did well at school. He was directed into vocational studies and got passes in woodwork and metalwork, but not in English, Maths or any academic subject.

At the age of 15, he left school and worked in a series of factories doing work of varying interest and hazard. Now aged 41, his job involved supervising the preparation of baths of paint stripper into which medium-sized objects like doors or tables were dipped. He had some concerns about this, because management had told him that paint stripper was highly flammable and so he made sure that there were no naked flames in the area.

Despite his best intentions, a new member of staff sneaked into a corner for a smoke break. When a table was lowered into the paint stripper some of the chemical splashed outwards in the direction of the unknown smoker. It caught fire immediately and flashed back so that the entire tank of paint stripper exploded.

It took the firemen 5 minutes to reach the site and another 20 minutes to put out the flames. They retrieved Dave and sent him by blue light ambulance to the hospital because of his extensive burns and because of the damage done to his lungs by inhaling hot air.

More than 30% of his body was burned, so he was admitted to the intensive care unit. His damaged cells released the chemical messengers called cytokines that did a series of bad things. One was to damage his lungs; the second was to awaken stealth virus from the sanctuary sites where it had lain since his childhood.

Normally, it takes decades for the stealth virus to gain the upper hand with the immune system as it did eventually with Edith Morris. But the same sort of process can occur in younger people who experience sudden severe shocks such as a heart attack, a stroke, a road traffic accident or severe burns. This does not happen in every seropositive person, but does occur in about a third of them. Dave was a member of that unlucky third. Suddenly, his immune system was stunned and could not perform its important task of keeping the stealth virus suppressed. Within three days, stealth virus reactivated and appeared in his blood with a rapidly increasing viral load. The doctors did not know this, because no intensive care unit routinely tested for this virus. As the stealth virus replicated, it stimulated cells to release more cytokines that went on to damage his lungs even further.

Dave was put on a ventilator to help him breathe. His wife was shocked to see her previously fit and healthy husband reduced to a state of helplessness. The doctors had to sedate him to stop him fighting against the ventilator and had to give him powerful painkillers. They were always guarded when they discussed his prognosis, telling her that every day he survived was a good sign. She spent most of her time sitting by his bedside, just in case he improved enough to be aware of her existence.

After three weeks, his immune system started to gain control of the stealth virus again, so the amount of cytokines declined. The doctors did not know this, because the tests required are found only in research labs. Instead, they observed his reduced need for oxygen in the ventilator and so started to look a little more optimistic. After another week, they were able to wean him off the ventilator and stop the drugs which were sedating him so, at last, he could open his eyes and see his tearful wife. Over the next few days they moved him into a general ward and she explained what had happened to him.

Many people who need ventilation in the intensive care unit do not survive the experience, but Dave was one of the fortunate ones. He went home after 60 days in the hospital, 48 of them spent in intensive care. When the doctors coded his reasons for admission, nobody mentioned that the stealth virus had lengthened his hospital stay, because nobody knew that this had happened. If they had done so, they would have found that about 10% of all the days spent in intensive care units were attributable to reactivation of the stealth virus. Nobody gave him the antiviral drug that had helped Kate, because nobody knew that he had this infection.

Medical researchers, noting the increasing requirement for beds in intensive care able to provide ventilatory support, redoubled their efforts to develop better ventilator systems which people could tolerate for weeks and even months. They did not attempt to inhibit the effect of stealth virus on the lungs despite the fact that this was one of the causes of the increasing demand.

Chapter 17: 2009-2011

2009 was another landmark year for the Alabama researchers.

First, Bob Pass obtained the results from his vaccine study in women of childbearing age. Seronegative women had been identified on the postnatal wards and encouraged to enter the study. They were randomised to receive three doses of glycoprotein B vaccine plus adjuvant or to receive 3 doses of placebo. They were followed closely to detect primary infection by testing on 17 occasions to measure viral load in blood, urine and vaginal secretions. Bob hoped that this close monitoring would show that the vaccine decreased either the duration of excretion of CMV or the viral load as a measure of success. However, the primary endpoint was the ability of the vaccine to protect women against acquiring primary CMV infection and this is what the Data Safety Monitoring Board members were keeping track of. Their aim was to ensure the safety of the volunteers in the study and its scientific integrity by stopping it early if there was evidence of toxicity or if it had proven its predetermined efficacy target. As planned, they met on two occasions to review the results before the study was due to finish. At the second of these meetings, they decided that the study should stop, because it had demonstrated approximately 50% protection against acquiring primary CMV infection. The results were so important that the study should stop early to allow these investigators, and others, to accelerate the evaluation of vaccines against CMV.

Bob's paper, published in the *New England Journal of Medicine*, clearly refuted the zeitgeist that it would be impossible to make vaccines against CMV. Some critical reviewers still commented that the efficacy was *only 50%*, ignoring the fact that the calculation by Paul and the CDC of the basic reproductive number had shown that this was nearly sufficient to eliminate CMV from a community by means of herd immunity. This criticism also ignored the fact that those working on HIV vaccines would be delighted with 50% efficacy against that virus. Clearly, reviewers were biased against CMV as a vaccine target and were using these comments of a political nature to come to conclusions instead of making decisions based on the scientific data. They were acting like revisionist historians, selecting particular pieces of information to support their preconceived ideas.

Second, David Kimberlin and Rich began their study of valganciclovir. Just as Rich had done when investigating herpes simplex encephalitis, all patients had to be given the standard of care, which was now ganciclovir for six weeks. They decided to do this by giving valganciclovir to all babies with congenital CMV in the study. They would then be randomised to complete six months of therapy with either valganciclovir or a matching placebo. In contrast to the initial study of six weeks of intravenous ganciclovir, a placebo could now be used because the drug was being given orally. Paul and Mike Sharland in London had accepted the offer to recruit patients into the study to get the answer more quickly, but neither of them would have believed how the clinical trials bureaucracy on both sides of the Atlantic could conspire to limit recruitment from the UK to only two cases out of the 104 needed. This was nothing to do with patient safety but was simply an example of the difficulties of transatlantic collaboration, because the two countries were divided by their common language as far as the regulatory authorities were concerned.

The white swan boats paddled slowly across the lake as this corner of Boston Common was taken over by those attending the 12th international CMV workshop organised by Theresa Compton in May 2009. Researchers from Germany announced that they had created a web based link which would allow people anywhere in the world to type in the sequence of two genes of CMV and determine if their local strain was resistant to ganciclovir or foscarnet.

In 2010, Bill and Suresh at last got results from another population which confirmed that many cases of congenital infection were due to reinfection of the mother. Virtually all women in Brazil are seropositive, so very few babies acquire CMV from primary infection of their mothers. The researchers monitored over 7,000 women, showed that many made new antibodies against glycoprotein H during pregnancy, and that this marker of reinfection with a new strain of CMV increased their risk of having a baby with congenital infection. They published their results in the *American Journal of Obstetrics and*

Gynecology to emphasise the need for a vaccine able to protect against multiple strains of CMV.

Sheila Dollard at the CDC in Atlanta reviewed the possibilities of screening dried blood spots by PCR as a means of diagnosing congenital CMV infection. The sensitivity was likely to be less than 100% for detecting infection, but might be higher for clinical cases, because babies who develop symptoms are more likely to have CMV detectable in their blood. Dried blood spots were thus potentially useful for identifying cases and offering them treatment, but large clinical trials would be needed to assess how this would perform in the real world.

Situated just 150 miles to the west of Atlanta, Suresh was disappointed when he saw the results of such a real-world study at the beginning of the year. Everyone agreed that it was important to conduct a large study to determine how testing dried blood spots for CMV DNA would work out in practice. Suresh and Karen Fowler had organised a massive study where samples from over 20,000 neonates were tested by PCR on blood and the standard DEAFF test on saliva. The results showed that testing dried blood spots detected only 34% of the cases of congenital CMV infection. It remained possible that more babies destined to develop symptoms had been identified because they had higher viral loads and were more likely to have viraemia, but the investigators would have to wait a few years before these results became available. Meanwhile, the results in front of them now did not seem encouraging for the prospects of persuading people to start screening for congenital CMV. It was not clear why some groups had very high sensitivity (100% in Italy) so an exchange of samples and lab protocols was warranted. It was also possible that the selection of particular patients for study had biased the earlier results towards those likely to have a higher viral load who would then be easier to detect by PCR.

However, Suresh was delighted at the end of the year to see the results of screening saliva swabs taken from neonates. 35,000 babies had been tested, half by one method and half by another. Overall, there was excellent agreement with the standard DEAFF test used on saliva, with virtually 100% of cases detected. The results were published in the *New England Journal of Medicine*. The lab methods had particularly been designed to be suitable for high throughput automation, so a candidate screening test for congenital CMV infection had at last been identified.

Maribavir offered the real potential of controlling CMV infection without poisoning the newly grafted bone marrow following transplantation. The results from the first study had been encouraging, but the choice of biomarkers for the definitive study after bone marrow transplantation was not propitious. Researchers knowledgeable about CMV had advised the drug company to choose the appearance of viraemia requiring preemptive therapy as the main endpoint for their study, to choose the highest of the three doses available and to give the drug soon after transplant instead of waiting for engraftment as was done for ganciclovir because of its bone marrow toxicity. None of these recommendations had been incorporated into the study design, partly because the regulatory agency wanted to see CMV disease as the main endpoint. The motivation of the regulators was to licence drugs only if they produced a real benefit for patients, not if they merely changed a value measured by a blood test. This was a laudable objective in general, but was misplaced for CMV because all patients were nowadays monitored for viraemia and given preemptive therapy if necessary. The effects of the placebo-controlled evaluation of the new drug would thus be masked by preemptive therapy in the way that belts and braces can both hold up trousers so that the effect of one cannot be assessed in the presence of the other.

When the code was broken, Michael Boeckh looked at the results and saw that there was no significant difference in CMV disease between patients who had received maribavir or placebo. The researchers from around the world, including Per Ljungman in Stockholm, had put a lot of effort into the study, but could only conclude that careful choice of biomarkers will be essential for future studies if other drugs against CMV with promising safety profiles are not to be lost to clinical practice.

The 13th international CMV workshop provided an opportunity to be educated about European history, for the organisers had hired the German National Museum in Nuremberg as the venue in May 2011.

Maria-Grazio Revello educated the audience about which women with primary CMV infection were at risk of transmitting virus to their fetus. She compared the ability of multiple diagnostic assays to discriminate between pregnant women who did or did not transmit virus. Overall, none of the assays performed well, showing that improved tests were required.

Clinical researchers in the UK were pleased to hear that a report by the Academy of Medical Sciences deemed the current regime of clinical trials regulation *not fit for purpose* and were delighted when the rules were to be replaced with a streamlined version. They hoped this would significantly accelerate planned studies to apply CMV biomarkers to clinical trial design. This included another joint study with Alabama and Mike Sharland in London to recruit babies aged 1 month to 4 years with both hearing loss and CMV, randomise them to valganciclovir for six weeks or matching placebo and see if progression of hearing loss could be altered in parallel with control of CMV viral load. If so, this would be the first treatment able to alter any cause of sensorineural hearing loss. Medical audiologists explained that they spent their lives identifying the precise cause of this hearing loss from among a multitude of possibilities, but that their interventions were limited to prescribing hearing aids or cochlear implants plus giving genetic counselling about the risk for a future sibling. If it became possible to reduce progression of hearing loss, that would be an important medical advance. In addition, it would have profound benefits for parents like Sue Rogers who might not have lost her home and her husband if progressive damage caused by CMV could have been stopped in its tracks.

A research group in the USA reported the results of a clinical trial which had used the excess of CD8 T-lymphocytes found in AIDS patients as a biomarker. They randomly allocated patients to receive valganciclovir for 8 weeks or a placebo and saw that the excess of CD8 T-lymphocytes in the blood of those given the drug declined slowly. This meant that CMV was driving the persistence of these cells so that this was a plausible mechanism for the cofactor effect of CMV which had been ignored for decades and which had troubled Stevie Headbanger and Billy Rogers. Longer term studies would be required to see if this change translated into a clinical benefit for AIDS patients, but at least the subject was now being addressed. The results also suggested that the same phenomenon in the elderly, like Edith Morris, might also respond to valganciclovir, so that parallel studies of immunosenescence could be contemplated.

The researchers at the CDC put together the results from two different studies to answer an important question. They knew how many babies were born with congenital CMV each year. They could estimate how many women acquired primary CMV infection during the childbearing years and knew that only one third of them transmitted the virus across the placenta. They combined all of these results to show that only one in four babies acquired their congenital infection from mothers with primary infection. The remaining three in four cases were born to women who were immune before pregnancy. There was no way of calculating how many seropositive mothers had been reinfected with a different strain of CMV and how many had reactivated their own virus. However, it was clear that a vaccine able to prevent primary CMV infection in women would only prevent 25% of cases of congenital infection, albeit the most serious ones, when given to teenage girls. Also, the study emphasised that, while maternal immunity is not perfect at preventing transmission of virus across the placenta, it was effective at moderating the development of clinical problems in these babies, as was seen with Mary Simpson. What was needed now was a study to predict which babies born with congenital CMV infection would develop disease. The expectation was that many of those born to immune women would be protected from disease, especially if the mothers were just reactivating a latent infection that their immune systems had seen before.

Of course, giving a vaccine to toddlers at the same time as teenagers would also decrease the number of infections which transmitted to mothers and this could help to control primary CMV infection acquired in day care centres. In fact, Paul estimated that vaccination of toddlers would rapidly protect CMV seronegative women, especially if they learned more about this infection and decided to leave their children only with day care centres which required CMV vaccine to be given to children once it was licensed. Thus, informing women about their risks and options could interact with the availability of a vaccine to bring the worst form of congenital CMV infection under control rapidly.

Vaccination of toddlers would also decrease the number who reinfected their mothers, although this benefit would take longer to feed through into cases of congenital CMV, because seropositive women were exposed to other potential sources of CMV.

Finally, cases of congenital CMV caused by maternal reactivation would be the slowest to control, requiring girls vaccinated as toddlers or teenagers to enter the childbearing years before the number of cases declined. Fortunately, this was the type of maternal CMV infection least likely to damage the fetus, so vaccines might control CMV disease quicker than CMV infection. This was important information to show healthcare planners, for the development and introduction of a CMV vaccine would require long-term sustained commitment to controlling and then, ultimately, eliminating this infection, but might repay the investment even more rapidly than first imagined. Although these were just theoretical calculations, the possibility that a vaccine could be produced in the real world against CMV was about to receive a boost.

Once the code of the vaccine study was broken in London, it was clear that the glycoprotein B vaccine plus adjuvant was superior to placebo, having altered the viral load biomarkers post transplant. Paul's study in solid organ transplant candidates had achieved its objective of stimulating the development of CMV vaccines generally and, coming hard on the heels of Bob Pass' report in the *New England Journal of Medicine,* should stop any remaining grumblings that CMV vaccines would never be feasible. The protective immune response induced by the vaccine was antibody, which surprised many researchers who had assumed that induction of cell mediated immunity would be essential because, in these transplant patients, CMV disease occurred in the context of suppressed cell mediated immunity. The study also showed that naturally acquired immunity in seropositives could be boosted, exactly as had been described by Mike Oxman for VZV. Clinical studies of these two herpesviruses had proceeded hand-in-hand since Tom Weller had first isolated them both. Paul published the results in the *Lancet* and set about planning how large definitive studies could be conducted in transplant patients.

Soon after, Bob Pass published a paper showing that seropositive women of childbearing age could have their levels of antibody boosted by the glycoprotein B vaccine, so the stage was set for using vaccines to determine if the natural immune response to CMV could be rebalanced towards one better able to control CMV infection.

Subsequently, HIV researchers did a similar analysis on their prototype vaccines for that infection and showed that, contrary to assumptions, the protective element was antibody, not cell mediated immunity. If only they had paid more attention to CMV, they could have reached this conclusion earlier and accelerated development of a much-needed vaccine against HIV. CMV had been there at the beginning of the AIDS epidemic in 1981, had been reported to be a cofactor in 1989 and again in 2004, but nobody wanted to learn from this virus; instead, they wanted to reinvent the wheel. This example shows how scientific progress in one area can benefit another as long as researchers have an open mind, prepared to consider the possibilities offered without denying their relevance out of hand.

Another assumption made by CMV vaccine deniers was demolished in 2011. Reviewers always stated that CMV did not harm anyone unless they were immunocompromised and textbooks repeated this statement despite the absence of evidence. Paul always gave an analogy: one might observe that many people who smoked cigarettes appeared to be healthy, but only long-term follow-up could identify whether they ultimately suffered from their habit. The equivalent for CMV came from an analysis of the NHANES data set which had been used earlier by the CDC to confirm the calculations of the basic reproductive number for CMV and show that immunisation of only 50% of the population could lead to eradication of this virus.

Because CMV had been associated with accelerated atherosclerosis after heart transplant (one of Bob Rubin's indirect effects), a group of statisticians examined over 14,000 people from the general population who had CMV antibodies measured as well as C reactive protein, a marker for atherosclerosis. They showed that mortality was strongly linked to CMV and that the association persisted after controlling for a variety of variables such as smoking and obesity. The effect of CMV was independent of C reactive protein, but the magnitude of the CMV effect was similar to that of C reactive protein. Because the latter was already accepted as a population level marker of mortality, this demonstrated that CMV could also be used for this purpose. To put the CMV effect another way, those who were CMV seropositive lived for approximately one year less on average than did those who were seronegative. Whether this was the result of CMV associated immunosenescence (as seen with Edith Morris) remained to be determined.

Importantly, this study also rejected another criticism which had been made about CMV vaccines, without any evidence to back it up. Commentators had questioned the ethics of giving a CMV vaccine to both boys and girls. They accepted that CMV caused problems during pregnancy, but assumed that administration to boys would not give them any direct benefit. This opinion assumed that boys had no interest in being the fathers of babies whose hearing had not been damaged. It also ignored the precedent of rubella vaccine which was routinely given to all children in order to interrupt transmission to women of childbearing age. Nevertheless, this opinion had been influential in the past and could now be rejected because males would expect to live longer if they avoided CMV by means of vaccination. Furthermore, CMV affected transplant patients and those with AIDS. While the former were about 50% male and 50% female, the majority of people with AIDS were male. Thus, there was another reason for CMV vaccine to be given routinely to children of both sexes, especially as it should be able to control the other occasions when CMV could damage people who were not in the major risk groups of pregnancy, transplant or AIDS patients.

Richard Davis was thin and pale. Although he was only 24, he had endured ulcerative colitis for 8 years now and had been admitted to hospital four separate times with relapses. On each occasion, he had fever and diarrhoea which responded slowly to treatment with steroids.

His fifth attack started while he was at work. Offering his apologies to his supervisor, he went straight to the hospital. The diagnostic skills of the junior doctor were not challenged, given Richard's history, so he started his new patient on a course of steroids to treat what he thought was a typical recurrence of ulcerative colitis.

Richard knew that it would be a few days before he felt better, but time dragged on and he still had a high fever and profuse diarrhoea. The doctors wondered if he had a bacterial infection, but all the cultures were negative. They gave him more steroids to dampen down the inflammation.

Richard's high fever did not respond and he became more and more toxic. The doctors were increasingly concerned and asked their surgical colleagues for advice. Occasionally, it was necessary to remove the patient's colon to save their life.

The surgeons advised close monitoring of his temperature, pulse, blood pressure and blood biomarkers of inflammation. All of these continued to deteriorate, so they decided to operate just as Richard was on the verge of delirium. The surgery was a success, Richard survived, his toxic state resolved, his fever disappeared and he looked much better. After a few days, he learned about his new colostomy and how he would need to care for it. He was disappointed and a little embarrassed to have this protuberance on his tummy, but was relieved not to have that terrible fever any more. After a week, he was fit enough to return home for convalescence.

Two weeks later, the histopathologists issued their report on the colon. It was riddled with inclusion bodies typical of stealth virus.

The doctors tested blood from Richard and confirmed that he had primary infection. They met to review the case and resolved there and then to always investigate patients who appeared to have a recurrence of ulcerative colitis for the possibility that they might have stealth virus instead. The junior doctor's diagnostic skills had been challenged, because a first episode of stealth virus infection in these patients given steroids looked just like a relapse of ulcerative colitis. Treatment with ganciclovir and avoidance of steroids might have allowed Richard to keep his colon and avoid the colostomy.

Stealth virus did not just cause disease in pregnant women and the immunocompromised; lots of people would benefit if this virus could be brought under control.

Chapter 18:
2012

At the close of the Civil War, which Paul had been told was the *War of Northern Aggression*, medical textbooks had been collected and brought back to Washington, DC to be stored in the Riggs Bank building. When Abraham Lincoln was assassinated in 1865 during a play called "Our American Cousins," the public demanded that Ford's Theatre be closed. The following year, the government purchased the empty theatre and used it to store the increasing number of medical books. This site flourished and the *Index Medicus* was created to keep track of inventory. In 1956, the establishment was named the National Library of Medicine with plans to move it to the campus of the National Institutes of Health. The driving force behind this proposed move was provided by two senators; John Fitzgerald Kennedy and Lister Hill. The National Library of Medicine opened at its new and still current site in 1962 while JFK was president and the main auditorium was named after Lister Hill.

In 2012, the Lister Hill auditorium was the location for a two-day public meeting organised jointly by the Food and Drug Administration, the National Institutes of Health, the

Centers for Disease Control and Prevention and the National Vaccine Program Office. The objective was to seek agreement about the developmental programme for vaccines against cytomegalovirus.

Once the discussions were underway, it became clear that the consensus concerning the prospects of making vaccines against CMV had moved from *impossible* to *likely*. Nothing had altered scientifically to effect this change; there had been no breakthrough discovery of a new lab technique, a new concept in immunology or a new way of making vaccines. Instead, thanks to the year 2000 report from the Institute of Medicine, investigators had been allowed to conduct clinical trials of vaccines which had been gathering dust on shelves for years. And the results had been very encouraging! In addition to the studies reported by Bob and Paul of glycoprotein B vaccine, another study was published in the week that the experts met in the Lister Hill Auditorium. This vaccine was different, because it aimed to stimulate cell mediated immunity as well as humoral immunity and had been given to bone marrow transplant patients with clear evidence of a beneficial effect. The researchers had started by giving the vaccine to the donor of the bone marrow in order to transfer immunity into the recipient, but had abandoned this aspect because most donors nowadays came from unrelated altruists living miles away, often in other countries, rather than from accessible siblings. Nevertheless, the study had continued with administration of vaccine to recipients only.

Three clinical trials of CMV vaccines had been conducted recently and all gave positive results. These findings cancelled the effect of the same old reviewers acting like revisionist historians, trying to make the facts fit their preconceived ideas by declaring that CMV vaccines were impossible to make. Instead of claiming to understand this complex infection and its multiple diseases, they should have allowed the standard scientific process to address the problem; state a hypothesis, design a study to address it and learn from the results.

The remaining uncertainty about the precise design of the large clinical trials which would be required for licensure was discussed and debated. At the end of the second day, there was a clear consensus on how to proceed. Provided that detailed case definitions could be produced, several pharmaceutical companies indicated that they were ready to apply their expertise in vaccine development to address the problem of CMV. It was hoped that one or more of their products would make CMV a vaccine-preventable infection in neonates, pregnant women and transplant patients. 2012 was a fitting time for this change in heart about the prospects for making CMV vaccines, for it was exactly 20 years since Martha Yow's impassioned plea in her *New England Journal of Medicine* editorial: ***we should not wait another 20 years, while thousands of additional children are born seriously handicapped.***

Some vaccines would aim to stimulate more potent antibodies, some would stimulate cell-mediated immunity while some would do both simultaneously in a single preparation. Nobody could predict which would be most successful, but several of these vaccines may well be able to control CMV sufficiently to allow herd immunity to complete the job and eliminate this infection from developed countries. Whether they could go further and eradicate CMV from the globe would be a question for a future generation but, to personify CMV, it should be quaking in its shoes at this moment, because this was clearly the beginning of the end.

Author's note

The case histories given here represent authentically the heartache and suffering that CMV can bring to people and their families. The names of the patients have been changed (except, of course, in the case of the Pope). After decades of counselling pregnant women with CMV infection about their individual risks of having a baby damaged by this virus, I still have difficulty answering their questions such as: why haven't I heard about this infection before? Why wasn't I told about this risk by my family doctor or antenatal clinic? Why wasn't I given a vaccine against such a common and important infection? This failure to identify CMV as an important pathogen worthy of control by immunisation cannot be described as a conspiracy of silence, because that implies an active process; instead, the subject has suffered from benign neglect. Many people have ignored CMV simply because it does not often produce overt symptoms to declare its presence. In this way, it can be thought of as flying below the radar used by doctors and scientists to identify important pathogens; hence the name, *Stealth Virus*.

In writing this book I identified the key papers which helped take CMV from an obscure infection to one that can be treated with antiviral agents and which will shortly be preventable by means of vaccination. To avoid introducing too many characters, I mentioned by name only those who appeared more than once. I also used their name to represent the whole research team which made each discovery and list below the authors of the relevant publications. I did not want to interupt the flow of the narrative by citing these references to support each substantive statement, in the style used by scientific texts. Instead, I grouped the references together in this last section according to the chapter where they were first mentioned. These references are key, but represent only a tiny proportion of the published scientific investigation into CMV, so I apologise to the many colleagues whose work has not been cited.

Many of the investigators named have committed their whole professional working lives to studying CMV. They have done this in a collegiate manner, exchanging reagents and laboratory protocols as well as inviting staff to visit to learn new techniques and return to their home laboratories. The whole subject of CMV is so huge that many research groups focused on their specialties; paediatrics in Alabama, pregnant women in Italy, solid organ transplant patients in London and Boston, bone marrow transplant patients in Seattle, AIDS patients in London and San Diego, vaccine development in Philadelphia, Alabama and London. In reviewing the key papers, I could not identify a single example where results from an experiment in mice helped move the subject forward. Those experiments provide fascinating examples of cutting-edge science and illustrate the evolution of the murine virus with its host, but I question whether this can be described as a model of human disease caused by human CMV.

The whole international effort to bring CMV under control has been hampered by bureacracy and by reviewers determined to make CMV fit neatly into their textbook chapter about rubella. Even in 2012, there are still reviewers out there, acting like revisionist historians, trying to make the facts fit their preconceived ideas. They have held up the development of CMV vaccines in the past, but will not succeed now, because the whole field has momentum, supported by evidence in humans, not opinion, just as Tom Weller would have wanted.

References cited

Chapter 1

Smith AJ, Weidman F. Infection of a stillborn infant by an amebiform protozoön (entamœba mortinatalium, *N.S.*). University of Pennsylvania Medical Bulletin 1910;23:285-98.

Chapter 2

Weller TH, Enders JF. Production of hemagglutinin by mumps and influenza A viruses in suspended cell tissue cultures. Proc Soc Exp Biol Med 1948 Oct;69(1):124-8.

Enders JF, Weller TH, Robbins FC. Cultivation of the Lansing Strain of Poliomyelitis Virus in Cultures of Various Human Embryonic Tissues. Science 1949 Jan 28;109(2822):85-7.

Weller TH. Serial propagation in vitro of agents producing inclusion bodies derived from varicella and herpes zoster. Proc Soc Exp Biol Med 1953 Jun;83(2):340-6.

Weller TH, Macauley JC, Craig JM, Wirth P. Isolation of intranuclear inclusion producing agents from infants with illnesses resembling cytomegalic inclusion disease. Proc Soc Exp Biol Med 1957 Jan;94(1):4-12.

Weller TH, Alford CA, Jr., NEVA FA. Retrospective diagnosis by serologic means of congenitally acquired rubella infections. N Engl J Med 1964 May 14;270:1039-41.

Hill RB, Jr., Rowlands DT, Jr., Rifkind D. Infectious pulmonary disease in patients receiving immunosuppressive therapy for organ transplantation. N Engl J Med 1964 Nov 12;271:1021-7.

Chapter 3

Klemola E, Kaariainen L. Cytomegalovirus as a possible cause of a disease resembling infectious mononucleosis. Br Med J 1965 November 6;2(5470):1099-102.

Kaariainen L, Klemola E, Paloheimo J. Rise of cytomegalovirus antibodies in an infectious-mononucleosis-like syndrome after transfusion. Br Med J 1966 May 21;1(5498):1270-2.

Chapter 4

Weller TH. The cytomegaloviruses: ubiquitous agents with protean clinical manifestations. I. N Engl J Med 1971 Jul 22;285(4):203-14.

Weller TH. The cytomegaloviruses: ubiquitous agents with protean clinical manifestations. II. N Engl J Med 1971 Jul 29;285(5):267-74.

Takahashi M, Otsuka T, Okuno Y, Asano Y, Yazaki T. Live vaccine used to prevent the spread of varicella in children in hospital. Lancet 1974 Nov 30;2(7892):1288-90.

Stagno S, Reynolds DW, Tsiantos A, Fuccillo DA, Long W, Alford CA. Comparative serial virologic and serologic studies of symptomatic and subclinical congenitally and natally acquired cytomegalovirus infections. J Infect Dis 1975 Nov;132(5):568-77.

Stern H, Tucker SM. Prospective study of cytomegalovirus infection in pregnancy. Br Med J 1973 May 5;2(5861):268-70.

Griffiths PD, Campbell-Benzie A, Heath RB. A prospective study of primary cytomegalovirus infection in pregnant women. Br J Obstet Gynaecol 1980 Apr;87(4):308-14.

Chapter 5

Stagno S, Reynolds DW, Huang ES, Thames SD, Smith RJ, Alford CA. Congenital cytomegalovirus infection. N Engl J Med 1977 Jun 2;296(22):1254-8.

Whitley RJ, Soong SJ, Dolin R, Galasso GJ, Ch'ien LT, Alford CA. Adenine arabinoside therapy of biopsy-proved herpes simplex encephalitis. National Institute of Allergy and Infectious Diseases collaborative antiviral study. N Engl J Med 1977 Aug 11;297(6):289-94.

Yeager AS, Grumet FC, Hafleigh EB, Arvin AM, Bradley JS, Prober CG. Prevention of transfusion-acquired cytomegalovirus infections in newborn infants. *J Pediatr* 1981;98:281-87.

Whitley RJ, Nahmias AJ, Soong SJ, Galasso GG, Fleming CL, Alford CA. Vidarabine therapy of neonatal herpes simplex virus infection. Pediatrics 1980 Oct;66(4):495-501.

MMWR. Pneumocystis pneumonia--Los Angeles. MMWR Morb Mortal Wkly Rep 1981 Jun 5;30(21):250-2.

MMWR. Kaposi's sarcoma and Pneumocystis pneumonia among homosexual men--New York City and California. MMWR Morb Mortal Wkly Rep 1981 Jul 3;30(25):305-8.

Randy Shilts. *And the Band Played On: Politics, People, and the AIDS Epidemic*. St Martin's Press, 1987.

Chapter 6

Elion GB, Furman PA, Fyfe JA, de MP, Beauchamp L, Schaeffer HJ. Selectivity of action of an antiherpetic agent, 9-(2-hydroxyethoxymethyl) guanine. Proc Natl Acad Sci USA 1977 Dec;74(12):5716-20.

Stagno S, Pass RF, Dworsky ME, Henderson RE, Moore EG, Walton PD, et al. Congenital cytomegalovirus infection: The relative importance of primary and recurrent maternal infection. N Engl J Med 1982 Apr 22;306(16):945-9.

Chapter 7

Pass RF, Little EA, Stagno S, Britt WJ, Alford CA. Young children as a probable source of maternal and congenital cytomegalovirus infection. N Engl J Med 1987 May 28;316(22):1366-70.

Griffiths PD, Panjwani DD, Stirk PR, Ball MG, Ganczakowski M, Blacklock HA, et al. Rapid diagnosis of cytomegalovirus infection in immunocompromised patients by detection of early antigen fluorescent foci. Lancet 1984 Dec 1;2(8414):1242-5.

Chapter 8

Plotkin SA, Smiley ML, Friedman HM, Starr SE, Fleisher GR, Wlodaver C, et al. Towne-vaccine-induced prevention of cytomegalovirus disease after renal transplants. Lancet 1984 Mar 10;1(8376):528-30.

Whitley RJ, Alford CA, Hirsch MS, Schooley RT, Luby JP, Aoki FY, et al. Vidarabine versus acyclovir therapy in herpes simplex encephalitis. N Engl J Med 1986 Jan 16;314(3):144-9.

Treatment of serious cytomegalovirus infections with 9-(1,3-dihydroxy-2-propoxymethyl)guanine in patients with AIDS and other immunodeficiencies. Collaborative DHPG Treatment Study Group. N Engl J Med 1986 Mar 27;314(13):801-5.

Grundy JE, Lui SF, Super M, Berry NJ, Sweny P, Fernando ON, et al. Symptomatic cytomegalovirus infection in seropositive kidney recipients: reinfection with donor virus rather than reactivation of recipient virus. Lancet 1988 Jul 16;2(8603):132-5.

Chapter 9

Saiki RK, Gelfand DH, Stoffel S, Scharf SJ, Higuchi R, Horn GT, et al. Primer-directed enzymatic amplification of DNA with a thermostable DNA polymerase. Science 1988 Jan 29;239(4839):487-91.

Chapter 10

Rubin RH. The indirect effects of cytomegalovirus infection on the outcome of organ transplantation. JAMA 1989 Jun 23;261(24):3607-9.

Webster A, Lee CA, Cook DG, Grundy JE, Emery VC, Kernoff PB, et al. Cytomegalovirus infection and progression towards AIDS in haemophiliacs with human immunodeficiency virus infection. Lancet 1989 Jul 8;2(8654):63-6.

Rubin RH. Preemptive therapy in immunocompromised hosts. N Engl J Med 1991 Apr 11;324(15):1057-9.

Schmidt GM, Horak DA, Niland JC, Duncan SR, Forman SJ, Zaia JA. A randomized, controlled trial of prophylactic ganciclovir for cytomegalovirus pulmonary infection in recipients of allogeneic bone marrow transplants; The City of Hope-Stanford-Syntex CMV Study Group. N Engl J Med 1991 Apr 11;324(15):1005-11.

Fowler KB, Stagno S, Pass RF, Britt WJ, Boll TJ, Alford CA. The outcome of congenital cytomegalovirus infection in relation to maternal antibody status. N Engl J Med 1992 Mar 5;326(10):663-7.

Yow MD, Demmler GJ. Congenital cytomegalovirus disease--20 years is long enough. N Engl J Med 1992 Mar 5;326(10):702-3.

Fox JC, Griffiths PD, Emery VC. Quantification of human cytomegalovirus DNA using the polymerase chain reaction. J Gen Virol 1992 Sep;73 (Pt 9):2405-8.

Rabkin CS, Hatzakis A, Griffiths PD, Pillay D, Ragni MV, Hilgartner MW, et al. Cytomegalovirus infection and risk of AIDS in human immunodeficiency virus-infected hemophilia patients. National Cancer Institute Multicenter Hemophilia Cohort Study Group. J Infect Dis 1993 Nov;168(5):1260-3.

Pillay D, Lipman MC, Lee CA, Johnson MA, Griffiths PD, McLaughlin JE. A clinico-pathological audit of opportunistic viral infections in HIV- infected patients. AIDS 1993 Jul;7(7):969-74.

Chapter 11

Stagno S, Cloud GA. Working parents: the impact of day care and breast-feeding on cytomegalovirus infections in offspring. Proc Natl Acad Sci U S A 1994 Mar 29;91(7):2384-9.

Bratcher DF, Bourne N, Bravo FJ, Schleiss MR, Slaoui M, Myers MG, et al. Effect of passive antibody on congenital cytomegalovirus infection in guinea pigs. J Infect Dis 1995 Oct;172(4):944-50.

Adler SP, Starr SE, Plotkin SA, Hempfling SH, Buis J, Manning ML, et al. Immunity induced by primary human cytomegalovirus infection protects against secondary infection among women of childbearing age. J Infect Dis 1995 Jan;171(1):26-32.

Einsele H, Ehninger G, Hebart H, Wittkowski KM, Schuler U, Jahn G, et al. Polymerase chain reaction monitoring reduces the incidence of cytomegalovirus disease and the duration and side effects of antiviral therapy after bone marrow transplantation. Blood 1995 Oct 1;86(7):2815-20.

Cha TA, Tom E, Kemble GW, Duke GM, Mocarski ES, Spaete RR. Human cytomegalovirus clinical isolates carry at least 19 genes not found in laboratory strains. J Virol 1996 Jan;70(1):78-83.

Chapter 12

Bowen EF, Wilson P, Cope A, Sabin C, Griffiths P, Davey C, et al. Cytomegalovirus retinitis in AIDS patients: influence of cytomegaloviral load on response to ganciclovir, time to recurrence and survival. AIDS 1996 Nov;10(13):1515-20.

Whitley RJ, Cloud G, Gruber W, Storch GA, Demmler GJ, Jacobs RF, et al. Ganciclovir treatment of symptomatic congenital cytomegalovirus infection: results of a phase II study. National Institute of Allergy and Infectious Diseases Collaborative Antiviral Study Group. J Infect Dis 1997 May;175(5):1080-6.

Cope AV, Sweny P, Sabin C, Rees L, Griffiths PD, Emery VC. Quantity of cytomegalovirus viruria is a major risk factor for cytomegalovirus disease after renal transplantation. J Med Virol 1997 Jun;52(2):200-5.

Cope AV, Sabin C, Burroughs A, Rolles K, Griffiths PD, Emery VC. Interrelationships among quantity of human cytomegalovirus (HCMV) DNA in blood, donor-recipient serostatus, and administration of methylprednisolone as risk factors for HCMV disease following liver transplantation. J Infect Dis 1997 Dec;176(6):1484-90.

Spector SA, Hsia K, Crager M, Pilcher M, Cabral S, Stempien MJ. Cytomegalovirus (CMV) DNA load is an independent predictor of CMV disease and survival in advanced AIDS. J Virol 1999 Aug;73(8):7027-30.

Lazzarotto T, Spezzacatena P, Varani S, Gabrielli L, Pradelli P, Guerra B, et al. Anticytomegalovirus (anti-CMV) immunoglobulin G avidity in identification of pregnant women at risk of transmitting congenital CMV infection. Clin Diagn Lab Immunol 1999 Jan;6(1):127-9.

Lazzarotto T, Guerra B, Spezzacatena P, Varani S, Gabrielli L, Pradelli P, et al. Prenatal diagnosis of congenital cytomegalovirus infection. J Clin Micro 1998: 3540-4.

Revello MG, Sarasini A, Zavattoni M, Baldanti F, Gerna G. Improved prenatal diagnosis of congenital human cytomegalovirus infection by a modified nested polymerase chain reaction. J Med Virol 1998 Sep;56(1):99-103.

Revello MG, Percivalle E, Arbustini E, Pardi R, Sozzani S, Gerna G. In vitro generation of human cytomegalovirus pp65 antigenemia, viremia, and leukoDNAemia. J Clin Invest 1998 Jun 15;101(12):2686-92.

Pass RF, Duliege AM, Boppana S, Sekulovich R, Percell S, Britt W, et al. A subunit cytomegalovirus vaccine based on recombinant envelope glycoprotein B and a new adjuvant. J Infect Dis 1999 Oct;180(4):970-5.

Frey SE, Harrison C, Pass RF, Yang E, Boken D, Sekulovich RE, et al. Effects of antigen dose and immunization regimens on antibody responses to a cytomegalovirus glycoprotein B subunit vaccine. J Infect Dis 1999 Nov;180(5):1700-3.

Fowler KB, Dahle AJ, Boppana SB, Pass RF. Newborn hearing screening: will children with hearing loss caused by congenital cytomegalovirus infection be missed? J Pediatr 1999 Jul;135(1):60-4.

Boppana SB, Fowler KB, Britt WJ, Stagno S, Pass RF. Symptomatic congenital cytomegalovirus infection in infants born to mothers with preexisting immunity to cytomegalovirus. Pediatrics 1999 Jul;104(1 Pt 1):55-60.

Deayton J, Mocroft A, Wilson P, Emery VC, Johnson MA, Griffiths PD. Loss of cytomegalovirus (CMV) viraemia following highly active antiretroviral therapy in the absence of specific anti-CMV therapy. AIDS 1999 Jul 9;13(10):1203-6.

Looney RJ, Falsey A, Campbell D, Torres A, Kolassa J, Brower C, et al. Role of cytomegalovirus in the T cell changes seen in elderly individuals. Clin Immunol 1999 Feb;90(2):213-9.

Emery VC, Cope AV, Bowen EF, Gor D, Griffiths PD. The dynamics of human cytomegalovirus replication in vivo. J Exp Med 1999 Jul 19;190(2):177-82.

Emery VC, Sabin CA, Cope AV, Gor D, Hassan-Walker AF, Griffiths PD. Application of viral-load kinetics to identify patients who develop cytomegalovirus disease after transplantation. Lancet 2000 Jun 10;355(9220):2032-6.

Emery VC, Griffiths PD. Prediction of cytomegalovirus load and resistance patterns after antiviral chemotherapy. Proc Natl Acad Sci U S A 2000 Jul 5;97(14):8039-44.

Chapter 13

Griffiths PD, McLean A, Emery VC. Encouraging prospects for immunisation against primary cytomegalovirus infection. Vaccine 2001 Jan 8;19(11-12):1356-62.

Stratton KR, Durch JS, Lawrence RS. Vaccines for the 21st Century. Washington,DC.: National Academy Press. 2000.

Boppana SB, Rivera LB, Fowler KB, Mach M, Britt WJ. Intrauterine transmission of cytomegalovirus to infants of women with preconceptional immunity. N Engl J Med 2001 May 3;344(18):1366-71.

Bourne N, Schleiss MR, Bravo FJ, Bernstein DI. Preconception immunization with a cytomegalovirus (CMV) glycoprotein vaccine improves pregnancy outcome in a guinea pig model of congenital CMV infection. J Infect Dis 2001 Jan 1;183(1):59-64.

Revello MG, Baldanti F, Percivalle E, Sarasini A, De-Giuli L, Genini E, et al. In vitro selection of human cytomegalovirus variants unable to transfer virus and virus products from infected cells to polymorphonuclear leukocytes and to grow in endothelial cells. J Gen Virol 2001 Jun;82(Pt 6):1429-38.

Chapter 14

Khan N, Shariff N, Cobbold M, Bruton R, Ainsworth JA, Sinclair AJ, et al. Cytomegalovirus seropositivity drives the CD8 T cell repertoire toward greater clonality in healthy elderly individuals. J Immunol 2002 Aug 15;169(4):1984-92.

Emery VC, Hassan-Walker AF, Burroughs AK, Griffiths PD. Human cytomegalovirus (HCMV) replication dynamics in HCMV-naive and -experienced immunocompromised hosts. J Infect Dis 2002 Jun 15;185(12):1723-8.

Schleiss MR, Bourne N, Bernstein DI. Preconception vaccination with a glycoprotein B (gB) DNA vaccine protects against cytomegalovirus (CMV) transmission in the guinea pig model of congenital CMV infection. J Infect Dis 2003 Dec 15;188(12):1868-74.

Fowler KB, Stagno S, Pass RF. Maternal immunity and prevention of congenital cytomegalovirus infection. JAMA 2003 Feb 26;289(8):1008-11.

Kimberlin DW, Lin CY, Sanchez PJ, Demmler GJ, Dankner W, Shelton M, et al. Effect of ganciclovir therapy on hearing in symptomatic congenital cytomegalovirus disease involving the central nervous system: a randomized, controlled trial. J Pediatr 2003 Jul;143(1):16-25.

Chapter 15

Hahn G, Revello MG, Patrone M, Percivalle E, Campanini G, Sarasini A, et al. Human cytomegalovirus UL131-128 genes are indispensable for virus growth in endothelial cells and virus transfer to leukocytes. J Virol 2004 Sep;78(18):10023-33.

Schleiss MR, Bourne N, Stroup G, Bravo FJ, Jensen NJ, Bernstein DI. Protection against congenital cytomegalovirus infection and disease in guinea pigs, conferred by a purified recombinant glycoprotein B vaccine. J Infect Dis 2004 Apr 15;189(8):1374-81.

Fowler KB, Stagno S, Pass RF. Interval between births and risk of congenital cytomegalovirus infection. Clin Infect Dis 2004 Apr 1;38(7):1035-7.

Mattes FM, Hainsworth EG, Geretti AM, Nebbia G, Prentice G, Potter M, et al. A randomized, controlled trial comparing ganciclovir to ganciclovir plus foscarnet (each at half dose) for preemptive therapy of cytomegalovirus infection in transplant recipients. J Infect Dis 2004 Apr 15;189(8):1355-61.

Deayton JR, Prof Sabin CA, Johnson MA, Emery VC, Wilson P, Griffiths PD. Importance of cytomegalovirus viraemia in risk of disease progression and death in HIV-infected patients receiving highly active antiretroviral therapy. Lancet 2004 Jun 26;363(9427):2116-21.

Nguyen HQ, Jumaan AO, Seward JF. Decline in mortality due to varicella after implementation of varicella vaccination in the United States. N Engl J Med 2005 Feb 3;352(5):450-8.

Oxman MN, Levin MJ, Johnson GR, Schmader KE, Straus SE, Gelb LD, et al. A vaccine to prevent herpes zoster and postherpetic neuralgia in older adults. N Engl J Med 2005 Jun 2;352(22):2271-84.

Sylwester AW, Mitchell BL, Edgar JB, Taormina C, Pelte C, Ruchti F, et al. Broadly targeted human cytomegalovirus-specific CD4+ and CD8+ T cells dominate the memory compartments of exposed subjects. J Exp Med 2005 Sep 5;202(5):673-85.

Cannon MJ, Davis KF. Washing our hands of the congenital cytomegalovirus disease epidemic. BMC Public Health 2005;5:70.

Bradford RD, Cloud G, Lakeman AD, Boppana S, Kimberlin DW, Jacobs R, et al. Detection of cytomegalovirus (CMV) DNA by polymerase chain reaction is associated with hearing loss in newborns with symptomatic congenital CMV infection involving the central nervous system. J Infect Dis 2005 Jan 15;191(2):227-33.

Chapter 16

Barbi M, Binda S, Caroppo S. Diagnosis of congenital CMV infection via dried blood spots. Rev Med Virol 2006 Nov;16(6):385-92.

Jeon J, Victor M, Adler SP, Arwady A, Demmler G, Fowler K, et al. Knowledge and awareness of congenital cytomegalovirus among women. Infect Dis Obstet Gynecol 2006;2006:1-7.

Guerra B, Simonazzi G, Banfi A, Lazzarotto T, Farina A, Lanari M, et al. Impact of diagnostic and confirmatory tests and prenatal counseling on the rate of pregnancy termination among women with positive cytomegalovirus immunoglobulin M antibody titers. Am J Obstet Gynecol 2007 Mar;196(3):221-6.

Dollard SC, Grosse SD, Ross DS. New estimates of the prevalence of neurological and sensory sequelae and mortality associated with congenital cytomegalovirus infection. Rev Med Virol 2007 Sep;17(5):355-63.

Colugnati FA, Staras SA, Dollard SC, Cannon MJ. Incidence of cytomegalovirus infection among the general population and pregnant women in the United States. BMC Infect Dis 2007;7:71.

Walter S, Atkinson C, Sharland M, Rice P, Raglan E, Emery VC, et al. Congenital cytomegalovirus: Association between dried blood spot viral load and hearing loss. Arch Dis Child Fetal Neonatal Ed 2008 Jan 7;93(4):280-5.

Kimberlin DW, Acosta EP, Sanchez PJ, Sood S, Agrawal V, Homans J, et al. Pharmacokinetic and pharmacodynamic assessment of oral valganciclovir in the treatment of symptomatic congenital cytomegalovirus disease. J Infect Dis 2008 Mar 15;197(6):836-45.

Winston DJ, Young JA, Pullarkat V, Papanicolaou GA, Vij R, Vance E, et al. Maribavir prophylaxis for prevention of cytomegalovirus infection in allogeneic stem-cell transplant recipients: a multicenter, randomized, double-blind, placebo-controlled, dose-ranging study. Blood 2008 Feb 19;111(11):5403-10.

Staras SA, Flanders WD, Dollard SC, Pass RF, McGowan JE, Jr., Cannon MJ. Influence of sexual activity on cytomegalovirus seroprevalence in the United States, 1988-1994. Sex Transm Dis 2008 May;35(5):472-9.

Chapter 17

Pass RF, Zhang C, Evans A, Simpson T, Andrews W, Huang ML, et al. Vaccine prevention of maternal cytomegalovirus infection. N Engl J Med 2009 Mar 19;360(12):1191-9.

Yamamoto AY, Mussi-Pinhata MM, Boppana SB, Novak Z, Wagatsuma VM, Oliveira PF, et al. Human cytomegalovirus reinfection is associated with intrauterine transmission in a highly cytomegalovirus-immune maternal population. Am J Obstet Gynecol 2010 Mar;202(3):297-8.

Dollard SC, Schleiss MR, Grosse SD. Public health and laboratory considerations regarding newborn screening for congenital cytomegalovirus. J Inherit Metab Dis 2010 Oct;33(Suppl 2):S249-S254.

Boppana SB, Ross SA, Novak Z, Shimamura M, Tolan RW, Jr., Palmer AL, et al. Dried blood spot real-time polymerase chain reaction assays to screen newborns for congenital cytomegalovirus infection. JAMA 2010 Apr 14;303(14):1375-82.

Boppana SB, Ross SA, Shimamura M, Palmer AL, Ahmed A, Michaels MG, et al. Saliva polymerase-chain-reaction assay for cytomegalovirus screening in newborns. N Engl J Med 2011 Jun 2;364(22):2111-8.

Marty FM, Ljungman P, Papanicolaou GA, Winston DJ, Chemaly RF, Strasfeld L, et al. Maribavir prophylaxis for prevention of cytomegalovirus disease in recipients of allogeneic stem-cell transplants: a phase 3, double-blind, placebo-controlled, randomised trial. Lancet Infect Dis 2011 Apr;11(4):284-92.

Wang C, Zhang X, Bialek S, Cannon MJ. Attribution of congenital cytomegalovirus infection to primary versus non-primary maternal infection. Clin Infect Dis 2011 Jan 15;52(2):e11-e13.

Hunt PW, Martin JN, Sinclair E et al. Valganciclovir reduces T cell activation in HIV-infected individuals with incomplete

CD4+ T cell recovery on antiretroviral therapy. *J Infect Dis* 2011;203:1474-83.

Griffiths PD, Stanton A, McCarrell E, Smith C, Osman M, Harber M, et al. Cytomegalovirus glycoprotein-B vaccine with MF59 adjuvant in transplant recipients: a phase 2 randomised placebo-controlled trial. Lancet 2011 Apr 9;377(9773):1256-63.

Simanek AM, Dowd JB, Pawelec G, Melzer D, Dutta A, Aiello AE. Seropositivity to cytomegalovirus, inflammation, all-cause and cardiovascular disease-related mortality in the United States. PLoS ONE 2011;6(2):e16103.

Kharfan-Dabaja MA, Boeckh M, Wilck MB, Langston AA, Chu AH, Wloch MK, et al. A novel therapeutic cytomegalovirus DNA vaccine in allogeneic haemopoietic stem-cell transplantation: a randomised, double-blind, placebo-controlled, phase 2 trial. Lancet Infect Dis 2012 Jan 9.

Glossary of terms used

Academy of Medical Sciences:	An institution in the UK which elects eminent scientists who then consider and issue reports on contemporary medical problems
Acyclovir:	A licensed antiviral drug which inhibits HSV and VZV
Adaptive immunity:	A sophisticated type of immune response which recognises specific antigens of an infectious agent and can mount an enhanced response when antigen is seen again later due to the induction of memory
Adjuvant:	A chemical which produces an enhanced immune response to an antigen when incorporated into a vaccine
AIDS defining conditions:	A list of diseases which indicate that an affected patient is suffering from Acquired Immune Deficiency Syndrome

Amniocentesis:	Insertion of a needle through the abdominal wall of a pregnant woman to remove a sample of amniotic fluid for testing
Antibody:	A protein produced by a B-lymphocyte which can bind to and inactivate a virus particle
Antibody avidity test:	A blood test which determines whether antibodies have been made recently (low avidity) or whether they have been present for many months
Antigen:	A component of a protein in a virus or a vaccine against which an antibody is made
Antisera:	Serum samples taken from an animal which has produced antibodies against a virus given as a vaccine
Assay:	A laboratory test able to detect a virus or a component of a virus
Atypical lymphocytes:	White blood cells seen in the blood which may indicate a diagnosis of infectious mononucleosis
Avidity:	A laboratory assessment of how tightly an antibody binds to its antigen

Basic reproductive number:	A mathematical representation of the contagiousness of an infectious disease
Bicentennial:	The anniversary of an event which occurred 200 years previously
Biomarkers:	Changes in the results of laboratory tests which can be taken to indicate success of a given treatment or vaccination
B-lymphocyte:	A type of white blood cell which makes antibodies as part of the adaptive immune system
Bone marrow transplant:	A procedure where the diseased bone marrow of a recipient is replaced with that taken from a healthy donor
Burkitt's lymphoma:	A cancer of the lymph nodes found predominantly in children living in central Africa or Papua New Guinea
CD4 lymphocyte:	A form of white blood cell which helps other lymphocytes perform their function
CD8 T-lymphocyte:	A form of white blood cell which directly attacks cells in the body infected by a virus as part of adaptive immunity

CDC (Centers for Disease Control and Prevention):	A part of the federal government of the USA with responsibility for public health
Cell culture:	The technique of maintaining living cells in the laboratory so that they can be infected with a virus
Cell mediated immunity:	The type of adaptive immunity that is mediated directly by cells such as T-lymphocytes
Chickenpox:	A rash that is said to resemble chick-peas laid upon the skin
CMV (cytomegalovirus):	A member of the herpesvirus family which normally infects people without causing any symptoms a.k.a. the stealth virus
Cofactor:	A component of a disease process which enhances the activity of the primary agent causing the disease
Cold sores:	Small blisters on the lips which recur from time to time following reactivation of HSV
Congenital:	Present at birth
Contagious:	Able to transmit from one person to another

Controls:	Patients randomised to not receive an experimental treatment in order to define the natural history of the condition being studied during a clinical trial
C-reactive protein:	A protein which is released from the liver to appear in the blood as an indicator of active inflammation
Cytokine:	A chemical messenger
Cytopathic effect:	Characteristic changes in cultured cells seen under a light microscope which indicate that a virus is present
Day care centres:	Places provided for the provision of safe custody of children while their parents are at work
DEAFF:	A method for detecting CMV rapidly in cultured cells by means of a monoclonal antibody (Detection of Early Antigen Fluorescent Foci)
Dermatome:	A distinct patch of skin served by a single sensory nerve
Direct effects:	The consequences of CMV infection which are apparent in an individual

DNA (deoxyribonucleic acid):	A molecule which encodes information by means of the order in which its individual nucleosides are assembled; DNA is usually found in the nucleus of a cell
DNA polymerase enzymes:	Enzymes which take nucleosides and assemble them to form the polymer DNA
Double-stranded:	A form of DNA containing two separate but complementary strands
EBV (Epstein-Barr virus):	A herpesvirus which can cause infectious mononucleosis or Burkitt's lymphoma
Encephalitis:	Inflammation of the brain
Endpoint:	A predetermined objective of a clinical study
Epidemiologist:	A researcher who studies diseases in populations, such as epidemics
Experiment of medicine:	Demonstration of an important fact about biology by studying contemporary medical practice
Food and Drug Administration:	A part of the federal government of the USA which decides whether medicines are safe and effective enough to be sold to the public

Foscarnet:	A toxic antiviral drug sometimes used to treat CMV
Ganciclovir:	An antiviral drug with moderate toxicity that is usually used to treat CMV
Genes:	Stretches of DNA which direct the cell to make a particular protein
Genital herpes:	HSV infection of the genital area
German measles:	Common term for rubella
Glandular fever:	Common term for infectious mononucleosis
Glycoprotein:	A protein which has sugar attached; frequently found on the surface of cells and the surface of viruses
Glycoprotein B:	A glycoprotein on the surface of CMV which is a major target of antibodies which neutralise infectivity
Glycoprotein H:	A glycoprotein on the surface of CMV which is a target of antibodies which neutralise infectivity
Graft rejection:	A process involving T-lymphocytes and antibodies which recognise a transplanted organ as foreign and try to destroy it

Graft versus host disease:	A process caused by donor T-lymphocytes which recognise the patient as foreign and try to destroy him or her
Helper T lymphocytes:	Another name for CD4 lymphocytes
Histopathologists:	Doctors who make diagnoses by examining stained thin slices of tissue under a microscope.
HSV (herpes simplex virus):	A herpesvirus which causes cold sores, genital herpes and herpes encephalitis
HSV encephalitis:	Inflammation of the brain caused by infection with HSV
Humoral immunity:	The type of adaptive immunity which is mediated by antibodies
Immune evasion:	A process used by a virus to avoid the effects of the innate and adaptive immunity of the host
Immunocompromised host:	A patient whose immune system has been damaged
Immunoglobulin:	A concentrated form of the liquid part of peripheral blood from multiple blood donors which is rich in antibodies against a virus produced following natural infection

Immunosenescence:	A poorly defined term indicating that elderly people have inferior immune responses to those of young adults
Immunosuppressive drugs:	Chemicals given to deliberately damage the immune system in order to prevent graft rejection after transplantation
Immunotherapy:	Administration of a dose of vaccine to increase or improve an immune response among those who have already responded to natural infection with the particular virus
Inclusion bodies:	Characteristic swellings of cells seen by histopathologists in tissues taken from patients suffering from disease caused by CMV
Indirect effects:	The consequences of CMV infection which are not apparent in an individual but which can be seen in a population of patients
Infectious mononucleosis:	An illness characterised by fever, sore throat and fatigue where atypical lymphocytes are frequently found in the blood
Innate immunity:	A primitive, yet effective, system which recognises infectious agents by means of their general chemical make up and which does not exhibit memory

Institute of Medicine:	An institution in the USA which elects eminent scientists who then consider and issue reports on contemporary medical problems
Laboratory adapted strains:	Examples of viruses which are easier to grow in the laboratory than the wild-type found in patients
Latency:	A state of hibernation where herpes-virus DNA persists without producing any virus particles
Logarithm:	A way of presenting values on a graph where each number in the series 1, 2, 3, 4 represents 10, 100, 1,000, 10,000
March of Dimes:	A charity in the USA which funds medical research
Maribavir:	A drug active against CMV which has not been shown to be effective in clinical practice
Measles:	A virus infection which causes a rash and conjunctivitis
Medical virology:	A specialty concerned with the diagnosis, treatment and prevention of viruses of medical importance

Memory:	A characteristic of adaptive immunity which allows it to give an enhanced response to a specific antigen it has encountered previously
MMR:	A live attenuated vaccine providing protection against measles, mumps and rubella
Molecular biology:	A branch of science which functions at the level of individual molecules and their interactions
Monoclonal antibody:	The protein product of an individual B-lymphocyte
Multivariate analysis:	A statistical technique to identify which among a list of factors is primarily responsible for causing the disease under investigation
Mumps:	A virus infection which causes the salivary glands to swell
Naive lymphocytes:	White blood cells which have not yet committed themselves to search for a particular antigen
National Institutes of Health:	A part of the federal government of the USA with responsibility for funding medical research

National Vaccine Program Office:	A part of the federal government of the USA with responsibility for identifying vaccine preventable diseases
Natural history study:	An investigation in a cohort of patients to define when a virus is present in relation to their disease
NHANES (National Health and Nutrition Examination Survey):	A process of systematically sampling the whole USA population to provide a representative subgroup who can be examined for particular diseases or infections
Nucleic Acid:	A polymer constructed from individual monomers of nucleosides to form either DNA or RNA
Nucleoside:	A naturally occurring building block of DNA or RNA comprising a base linked to a sugar
Operation Desert Storm:	The military process of forcing Iraq to withdraw from Kuwait
Opportunistic infections:	A list of infectious agents which usually only cause disease in patients whose immune systems have been damaged
Pathogenesis:	The process by which an infectious agent causes disease

PCR (polymerase chain reaction):	A biochemical technique which uses DNA polymerase enzymes to amplify the amount of DNA found in a patient
Placebo:	A dummy medicine which looks and tastes like the real thing but which lacks the active ingredient
Placenta:	An organ found only in pregnant women which diverts nutrients to the fetus and removes metabolic breakdown products from the fetus
Poliovirus:	One of the three types of viruses which can cause poliomyelitis
Preemptive therapy:	The administration of an antiviral drug to a patient in whom CMV has been identified by a laboratory test with the intention of preventing disease
Primary infection:	The first time a patient's immune system has to respond to a particular virus
Primers:	Short stretches of linked nucleosides which bind to a template and direct a DNA polymerase enzyme where to start copying the template
Prodrug:	A pharmaceutical preparation given to a patient which is metabolised in the

	body to release a compound that has the desired therapeutic effect
Proteins:	Polymers made from a series of amino acids to create a large molecule which can perform specialised functions within a cell
Randomisation:	A process of minimising bias by allocating subjects to a treatment according to chance
Randomised:	A patient who has been allocated to one treatment instead of another
Reactivation:	The process by which a latent herpesvirus expresses the information within its hibernating DNA to produce infectious virus particles
Reinfection:	The process of initiating infection from without in an individual who has already been infected with a particular virus
Replication:	The process whereby a virus is copied within a cell to produce thousands of daughter viruses
RNA (ribonucleic acid):	A molecule which encodes information by means of the order in which its individual nucleosides are assembled; RNA

	is usually found within the cytoplasm of a cell
Rubella:	A virus infection which causes a rash and can damage the developing fetus
Sanctuary sites:	Cells within the body where CMV establishes itself by expressing its immune evasion genes to prevent the immune system gaining access
Sensorineural hearing loss:	A type of deafness caused when a virus destroys specialised cells within the structures of the inner ear
Seronegative:	A person lacking antibodies against a particular virus
Seropositive:	A person with antibodies against a particular virus
Shingles:	Common name for zoster, caused when VZV reactivates and infects an area of skin supplied by a single nerve
Single-stranded:	A form of DNA which is not accompanied by a complementary strand
Smallpox:	A disease with a characteristic rash which had a high mortality
Standard of care:	A combination of interventions which is generally considered by doctors to

	represent the best which can be delivered during contemporary medical practice
Strain:	A virus which differs slightly from others which bear the same name
Syndrome:	A characteristic constellation of symptoms and signs
Threshold value:	The quantity of viral load at which disease becomes very likely to occur
T-lymphocyte:	A type of white blood cell which functions in the adaptive immune system by directly killing virus-infected cells
Towne vaccine:	A prototype live attenuated vaccine against CMV
Vaccine:	A pharmaceutical product which presents antigens from a virus to the adaptive immune system to induce memory so that an enhanced response may be obtained when the patient encounters the real virus
Valganciclovir:	The prodrug of ganciclovir
Vidarabine:	An experimental antiviral drug which was not licensed
Viraemia:	The presence of virus in the blood

Viral load:	The quantity of virus found in the urine, saliva or blood
VZV (Varicella-Zoster virus):	A herpesvirus which causes chickenpox (varicella) and shingles (zoster)
Wild-type:	The form of a virus which is found in patients
Zoster:	A rash limited to a single dermatome which is caused by VZV reactivating and passing down a sensory nerve to infect the skin supplied by that nerve

6414173R00138

Printed in Great Britain
by Amazon.co.uk, Ltd.,
Marston Gate.